THE HAND

PRIMARY CARE OF COMMON PROBLEMS

SECOND EDITION

American Society for Surgery of the Hand
Hand Surgery Manuals Committee
Continuing Education Division

RICHARD S. IDLER, M.D., *Chairman*

RALPH T. MANKTELOW, M.D., *Council Liaison*

GEORGE LUCAS, M.D. *(Ex Officio)*

WILLIAM H. SEITZ, M.D.

DAVID C. BUSH, M.D.

MELVIN P. ROSENWASSER, M.D.

FRANK M. WATSON, JR., M.D.

MATTHEW D. PUTNAM, M.D.

DISCLAIMER

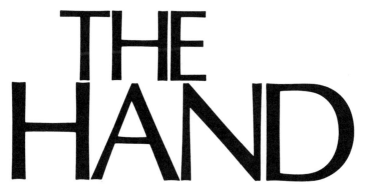

THE HAND

PRIMARY CARE OF COMMON PROBLEMS

AMERICAN SOCIETY FOR SURGERY OF THE HAND

SECOND EDITION

CHURCHILL LIVINGSTONE

A Division of Harcourt Brace & Company

NEW YORK, EDINBURGH, LONDON, PHILADELPHIA, SAN FRANCISCO

Library of Congress Cataloging-in-Publication Data

The Hand : primary care of common problems / American Society for
  Surgery of the Hand. — 2nd ed.
      p.   cm.
   Includes bibliographical references
   ISBN 0-443-08584-6
   1. Hand—Wounds and injuries—Surgery.   2. Hand—Surgery.
I. American Society for Surgery of the Hand.
   [DNLM: 1. Hand—Surgery.   2. Hand Injuries—therapy.   WE 830
H236]
RD559.H3594   1990
617.5'75—dc20
DNLM/DLC
for Library of Congress   89-70878
                                                                  CIP

Churchill Livingstone® is a registered trademark of Harcourt
Brace & Company.

 is a trademark of Harcourt Brace & Company.

Published and distributed in the United States by Churchill
Livingstone Inc., The Curtis Center, Independence Square West,
Philadelphia, PA 19106. Distributed in the United Kingdom by
Churchill Livingstone, Robert Stevenson House, 1–3 Baxter's Place,
Leith Walk, Edinburgh EH1 3AF, and by associated companies,
branches, and representatives throughout the world.

Accurate indications, adverse reactions, and dosage schedules for
drugs are provided in this book, but it is possible that they may
change. The reader is urged to review the package information data
of the manufacturers of the medications mentioned.

Acquisitions Editor: *Leslie Burgess*
Copy Editor: *Kamely Dahir*

Printed in the United States of America

9

FOREWORD

Many prominent teachers of hand surgery have made the observation over the years that the initial management of a patient with an injured hand will often have a crucial effect on the eventual outcome. In most instances, the patient with an injured hand is seen first by an emergency room physician, a house officer, a family practitioner, or paramedical personnel. By the same token, the initial recognition of nontraumatic hand disorders is usually made by a physician whose primary expertise is outside the realm of hand surgery.

With this in mind, the late Dr. Richard J. Smith saw the need for a concise, compact manual of hand surgery that might be used to disseminate knowledge of common hand disorders to this widely disparate group of physicians. Although input was sought and obtained from many members of the American Society for Surgery of the Hand, the initial manuscript was written by Dr. William L. Newmeyer, who did not attempt to write a definitive or comprehensive text on hand surgery, but rather to concentrate on procedures that fall within the purview of the office or emergency department.

As with most medical specialities, the treatment options for most hand injuries and disorders are wide and varied, and controversy abounds regarding the optimal treatment. However, by having the original manuscript reviewed by many members of the Hand Society, an attempt has been made to offer what is generally considered to be concensus management of the various disorders discussed in the text.

This book was revised for the second edition by Dr. Richard S. Idler and other members of the Hand Surgery Manuals Committee of the American Society for Surgery of the Hand. We are grateful to them for their efforts.

AMERICAN SOCIETY FOR SURGERY OF THE HAND
David P. Green, M.D.
President, 1988–89

PREFACE TO THE SECOND EDITION

Although in the course of recorded human history there has been little actual change in hand anatomy, our understanding of the hand's physiology and biomechanics has grown and will continue to do so. This knowledge, together with advances in surgical technique, has improved our ability to treat various injuries of the hand.

The first edition of this book provided an excellent source for information on management of basic injuries and other afflictions of the hand. This second edition has attempted to further refine these recommendations and to expand discussions on topics such as the wrist, where our understanding of injuries has grown considerably. Discussion has been kept brief, concise, and within the general consensus for examining and managing these problems.

As Chairman of the Hand Surgery Manuals Committee, I would like to thank my fellow members for their assistance in the revision of this text. We hope this re-

mains a helpful reference source for those who under-
take the care of hand injuries.

Richard S. Idler, M.D.
Chairman, Hand Surgery Manuals Committee, 1989

PREFACE TO THE FIRST EDITION

No book, article, TV cassette program, audio cassette program, or instructional course can provide the answer to every conceivable clinical situation. This volume is no exception. The material that follows is a consensus view of an approach to the primary management of common hand injuries and other commonly seen hand problems. It represents the thinking and experience of the committee members and of a number of other members of the American Society for Surgery of the Hand who reviewed the manuscript and made a number of helpful and useful suggestions.

Several caveats must be emphasized. There is no substitute for experience, hopefully under expert guidance. The saying, attributed to Simon Bolivar, that "good judgement comes from experience and experience comes from bad judgement," has a good deal of truth to it. It should always be remembered that there is no such thing as "a" or "the" method of treating a given problem. Successful methods in surgery are based on careful observation of and adherence to basic principles of management of diseased and injured tissue that include prevention of swelling, preservation of blood supply, control of hemorrhage, and immobilization of injured parts. Appropriate methods of treatment are built upon such principles and never contradict them.

Every physician treating patients with injuries and diseases of the hand should work within the boundaries of his knowledge and skills. Especially in treating hand injuries there is sometimes a temptation to push beyond those boundaries because life is seldom at stake. However, one should always remember that the patient's hand function and thus livelihood may well be at stake. Any physician who sees patients with hand injuries in an emergency setting should ask three questions: (1) should I treat the injury definitively here and now? or, (2) should I refer the patient for urgent treatment by a consultant either here or in an operating room? or, (3) can the definitive treatment of this patient's problem be safely postponed? If these questions are asked and honestly answered, the number of patients developing complications should be very small.

This volume is designed to be used in conjunction with *The Hand: Examination and Diagnosis* (written by a committee of the American Society for Surgery of the Hand, chaired by Richard Burton, M.D. and published in 1983 by Churchill Livingstone).* The reader will note that in some chapters examination and diagnosis seem to have been brushed over rather briefly. This is deliberate. If the reader will use the two volumes together, most traumatic and other hand problems can

---

* A third edition, updated by the Hand Surgery Manuals Committee, was published in 1990 by Churchill Livingstone Inc.

be accurately diagnosed and suitable primary treatment can be rapidly instituted.

Those persons most directly involved in the production of this book were the members of my committee who are listed elsewhere and who have my great thanks. Stephanie McCann turned our rough sketches into finished drawings and merits our gratitude. Dr. Richard Smith was the inspiration for this volume and a tireless and helpful editor through approximately eight revisions.

We hope that all readers find the book useful and interesting. Our sincere wish is that it will help to improve the primary care of patients with hand problems, thereby minimizing patient suffering and lowering the cost of both medical treatment and disability.

William L. Newmeyer, M.D.
Chairman, Office Procedures Manual Committee, 1985

ACKNOWLEDGMENTS

The concept of this book evolved in 1981 at a series of discussions initiated by the then vice president of the American Society for Surgery of the Hand, Dr. Richard Smith, with Dr. William Newmeyer, Dr. Gordon Mc-Farland, and myself. Because of Dr. Newmeyer's long-standing interest in teaching primary care physicians about the initial care of hand injuries and diseases, he willingly undertook the laborious task of chairing the ad hoc committee which has produced this find monograph. Each section of this monograph was developed by one of the committee members with suggestions coming from each of the other committee members. Dr. Newmeyer, in consultation with a number of members of the American Society for Surgery of the Hand, has worked long hours to edit and hone the monograph to its present state.

It is difficult to produce a brief manual which will be detailed enough to aid the general physician caring for the specific patient, and yet broad enough so as not to be constrictive of the many variables which any given condition may involve. The American Society for Surgery of the Hand does not mean to imply that these guidelines are the only ones, but merely common and currently used approaches to given hand problems. Obviously there are many acceptable alternatives which are not mentioned and new procedures and techniques continually become available.

The American Society for Surgery of the Hand is indebted to Dr. Newmeyer and his committee for their efforts in this task. Hopefully physicians involved in the primary care of patients with hand injuries and diseases will find value in these pages.

AMERICAN SOCIETY FOR SURGERY OF THE HAND
Richard I. Burton, M.D.
Coordinator, Division of Education, 1984

CONTENTS

1

GENERAL PRINCIPLES OF MANAGEMENT

URGENT CONSIDERATIONS

The first thing to do when seeing any patient with a hand injury is to make sure that there are no other serious life-threatening problems that demand urgent attention.

The only hand injury that is immediately life-threatening is one in which there is uncontrolled hemorrhage. This usually occurs when a major vessel is partially transected. If bleeding cannot be controlled by direct pressure, apply an arm tourniquet, exsanguinate the arm by elevation, and place pressure on the wound before inflating the cuff to 100 to 150 mmHg above systolic pressure. In almost all instances this will control hemorrhage in the hand. Very rarely it may be necessary to ligate a vessel, but great care must be taken to make sure that a structure other than the hemorrhaging vessel is not ligated. Specifically, one must make sure that a nerve is not accidentally ligated. One should never ligate a vessel if there is vascular compromise distally because repair of the vessel may be indicated, and this will be difficult or impossible if the vessel has been injured by a ligature. If the bleeding cannot be controlled in this fashion, the patient should be taken to the operating room at once.

Once bleeding is controlled and the patient's vital signs are stable, the examiner may proceed with a systematic evaluation of the patient's hand injury.Obviously, several things can be done at once, and the reader should keep that in mind in reading the ensuing paragraphs.

THE HISTORY

As with any other medical history one must evaluate not only the current problem but also pre-existing medical problems that may influence decisions about the care of the hand injury. Other medical problems, which appear unrelated to the hand, may have some bearing on the patient's management, especially if he requires a high regional or a general anesthetic for management of the hand injury. The examiner should be certain to inquire about medical problems such as diabetes, hypertension, heart disease, liver disease, coagulopathies, and pulmonary problems. All currently used medications should be noted, especially anticoagulant drugs. The time of the last ingestion of food or drink must be noted and, as a general rule, it is wise to make the patient NPO pending any decision about the need for surgery. A history of allergies, especially drug allergies, must be obtained as well as the current status of tetanus immunization. If the injury is from an animal bite, one must consider the possibility of rabies, the need for appropriate notification of public health authorities, and institution of treatment.

When asking about the hand injury, one should concentrate particularly on the mechanism of the current injury. How was the injury sustained? Was a tool involved? Was it a power or a hand tool? What was the magnitude of the forces involved? What position was the hand in when the injury occurred? What was the potential for contamination at the time of injury? One cannot get too much detail about the mechanism of injury. One should always note which hand is the dominant one. Record exactly which digit and which part of the digit, hand, or wrist was injured. If the chart is completed some time after the examination, it is not uncommon for the incorrect digit, surface, or hand to be noted in the medical record.

It is most important to get a history of any previous hand injuries. This is relevant for the immediate and subsequent management of the patient. It may also be very important if litigation is instituted at a later date. Often with a work related injury, workers' compensation payments and settlements may be greatly affected by the condition of the hand at the time of injury. In certain industries (e.g., sawmills) prior injuries are very common.

THE PHYSICAL EXAMINATION

The first step in any examination is to make the patient comfortable. With less severe injuries, he may be seated with the arm on a table. However, in most cases it is preferable for the patient to be supine on a stretcher or gurney. First, observe the hand in its resting position (Figs. 1 and 2). Next examine the hand for active function by having the patient put wrist and digits through as full a range of motion (ROM) as possible. Then gently palpate the hand to evaluate tender or swollen areas. Evaluate sensibility by stroking the area of potential loss with a cotton wisp or very gently touching it with a sterile fine needle and comparing the feeling in this area with that in a normal area.

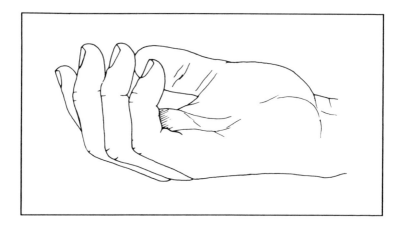

Figure 1
The normal quiescent hand with the forearm supinated showing increasing flexion tone of the digits from radial to ulnar

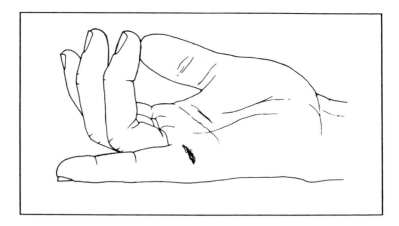

Figure 2
Typical attitude of a finger following division of both flexor tendons

The wound is then examined. *Warning*: If the injury is severe, and if immediate surgery is indicated, probing the wound in the emergency room may injure and contaminate tissues needlessly as well as disturbing the patient unnecessarily. In these cases leave the wound alone until the patient is anesthetized in the operating room.

The initial examination and treatment will often determine the ultimate success or failure of hand function. In the evaluation of an injury, check for the possibility of damage to important structures. With a deep laceration evaluate the function of structures lying distal to the wound. Severely angulated and rotated structures are gently realigned and supported on folded sterile towels or a splint to avoid further damage.

The following points are critical to note in examining and diagnosing the injured hand:

The skin

Any open injury involves the skin to some degree. Major skin loss obviously will require replacement. Sometimes this can be done in the outpatient setting but often it is more advisable to apply suitable dressings and delay the procedure. Small, innocuous appearing wounds can be accompanied by a significant amount of underlying damage. Be suspicious of deep structure injury and of the presence of a foreign body (or the remnant of a foreign body).

Vascular system

Signs of arterial insufficiency include pulselessness, pallor, pain, paresthesias, and paralysis. One can evaluate the patency of major arteries by the Allen test, as follows: Compress radial and ulnar arteries. Exsanguinate the hand by elevation or by having the patient rapidly flex and extend the fingers. Then alternately release the arteries to evaluate distal arterial filling. The blanched hand should "pink up" in 3 to 5 seconds if the artery being tested is patent. This test can also be applied to the digits. Rapid capillary filling in the presence of cyanosis and/or swelling indicates some venous obstruction that should be investigated.

Tendons

Observe the attitude of the hand and fingers at rest (see Figs. 1 and 2). Test for active function of the tendon system. One should always be aware of the possibility of partial lacerations of either flexor or extensor tendons. With flexor tendons, if one can observe a laceration of the tendon sheath, an effort should be made to observe the tendon as it goes through its normal glide.

With both flexors and extensors if no laceration or only a small nick is seen, nothing further needs to be done. If the laceration is over 30 percent to 40 percent of the tendon circumference, formal exploration and repair should be carried out. If one is not able to be quite certain about the extent of tendon injury, a formal exploration should be carried out.

Incomplete extension after a dorsal laceration usually indicates a complete extensor tendon laceration. In that case extension is accomplished by means of one of the bands (juncturae tendinium) interconnecting the extensor digitorum tendons on the back of the hand. Isolated injury to one of the bands is not of great functional importance.

Nerves

All nerves in the area of the wounds are considered injured unless tests prove them to be intact. Do not start the sensory examination with a sharp pin. This is particularly alarming to children (as well as to some adults). Gentle palpation of the area in question, comparing its sensibility to that of an uninjured part of the hand, will be helpful. Lack of sweat distal to the injury often is a telltale sign of sensory nerve injury. Pull a smooth metal object (such as a ball point pen barrel) across the digit. In a normal finger it will adhere to some extent because of the normal sweat. In a finger with a lacerated digital nerve it will not adhere. For mixed motor-sensory nerves evaluate motor function.

An alternative means for evaluating the sensory integrity of the nerves of the hand is the immersion or wrinkle test. Innervated glabrous skin will wrinkle after being immersed in water for 5 to 10 minutes. Localized failure of this phenomena suggests underlying nerve trauma.

Skeletal system

Displaced fractures and dislocations produce obvious deformity. Nondisplaced fractures and ligament injuries are more difficult to diagnose. With suspected bone or joint injury, palpate for localized tenderness. Joints should be stressed gently to test for instability or subluxation. A limited regional anesthetic can be used for stress testing.

DIAGNOSTIC TESTS

Radiographs

Radiographic examination is the most commonly used
and most important diagnostic test in evaluating the
injured hand. All injuries beyond the obviously superficial (e.g., sharp lacerations in which there is no suspicion of a foreign body) require radiographic examination.
One should never hesitate to be evaluated radiographically if there is any suspicion of a skeletal injury (new or
old) or a foreign body. As a general rule the only
radiograph a physician ever regrets is the one he did not
get. It is most important not to accept a verbal or written
report but always to view the radiographs yourself.

Special views that can be helpful include the following:

1. The clenched fist taken in the anteroposterior
   projection to assess possible intercarpal instability
   due to wrist ligament injury.
2. Xeroradiograms for relatively nonradiopaque foreign bodies.
3. The carpal tunnel view, which is taken with the
   wrist hyperextended and the x-ray beam aimed
   down the carpal canal. This can help to evaluate a
   possible hook of the hamate or pisiform fracture.
4. Tomograms may be helpful in detecting certain
   fractures (e.g., scaphoid fractures) that are suspected
   but not visible on routine views.
5. Oblique views and multiple views with the hand in
   different positions will sometimes reveal certain
   bone or joint problems not otherwise seen.
6. Comparison views (especially in children and in
   patients with wrist injuries) can reveal an injury by

contrasting the injured with the uninjured hand.
7. Stress views of a joint in the case of a suspected ligamentous injury can clinch a suspected diagnosis.
8. When ordering radiographs of digits be sure to get isolated laterals of them. Views in which four digits are superimposed upon one another are not very useful.
9. In some instances it is very helpful to use a C Arm (low radiation fluoroscopy) to monitor reduction of a fracture or removal of a foreign body on a video screen.

Wound culture

Older wounds, human and animal bites, and wounds sustained in badly contaminated areas should be cultured and Gram stains made and examined. Consider the possibility of obscure organisms (e.g., mycobacteria or fungi) and order the appropriate cultures.

Special diagnostic techniques

A Doppler flowmeter can be used to evaluate blood flow. In its simplest form this is a handheld device with earphones to listen to the blood flow. It may be used when it is difficult to palpate pulses.

A variety of other techniques can be used including radionuclide scans, devices to measure fascial compartment pressures, and the fluorescein dye test to gauge impending skin necrosis. These tests are generally not used in the outpatient setting.

Routine diagnostic tests

These tests include the usual preoperative studies tailored to the patient's age, medical condition, etc. In certain instances blood clotting studies and a sickle cell preparation may be indicated.

DETERMINATION OF THE SITE OF CARE

Following careful evaluation of the patient and injury, one should be prepared to provide definitive care in the most appropriate setting. A primary care physician should not try to do procedures or care for injuries that he does not feel comfortable handling. In many cases it is better to postpone definitive treatment if a consultant is not readily available.

The following conditions can often be handled comfortably in a well-equipped emergency room or outpatient surgery unit:

1. Nailbed lacerations or avulsions.
2. Finger pad amputations and other small skin avulsions which require no skin graft or only a small skin graft.
3. Superficial lacerations.
4. Superficial foreign bodies.
5. Simple closed fractures.
6. Extensor tendon injuries with easily retrieved tendon ends.
7. Localized infections.

The following injuries are usually better handled in a major operating room:

1. Finger pad amputations in which local or distant flaps are used.
2. Deep, extensive, or contaminated lacerations requiring exploration.
3. Many extensor tendon injuries.
4. Flexor tendon injuries.
5. Nerve injuries.
6. Deep foreign bodies.
7. Displaced, unstable, or irreducible fractures or dislocations.
8. Major crush injuries.
9. Deep infections.
10. Complex wounds and amputations.

EMERGENCY ROOM ATMOSPHERE

In the emergency room, the patient should be made as comfortable as possible in a supine position. Maintain a quiet and reassuring atmosphere to relieve patient anxiety. All constrictive clothing and jewelry should be removed. The judicious use of analgesics or sedatives will help minimize the patient's pain, but the patient should not be sedated to the point where he cannot leave after a simple procedure. Pain can also be lessened by continuous elevation and protective splinting. Avoid soaking the injured hand in an antiseptic solution while it is held in a dependent position. The treating physician should explain the problem as well as the necessary follow-up care and realistic prognosis for recovery from the injury to the patient.

When the hand is being treated (Fig. 3), the patient should be on a firm gurney, stretcher, or cot, with the hand placed on a stable platform at a height comfortable for the treating physician. There must be a good, adjustable light.

It is essential to have fine instruments in good condition to work on hand injuries. Castoffs and instruments that do not work will damage the tissues. The following is a basic set:

1. Small curved pointed scissors.
2. Fine, single tooth forceps.
3. A knife handle to take a # 15 blade.

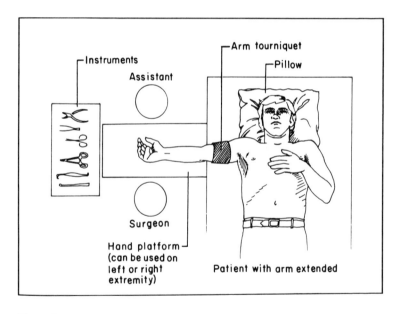

Figure 3
Diagram of the emergency room set up

4. Small suture scissors.
5. A small fine rongeur.
6. A small periosteal elevator.
7. Several mosquito clamps.
8. Two double prong skin hooks.
9. Two small right angle (Ragnell) retractors.
10. A Webster needle holder.

Some useful additions include these:

1. An irrigation set (a 10-ml syringe and a blunt 18-gauge needle serve well).
2. A battery operated coagulator.
3. A battery operated Kirschner- (K) wire inserter (or equivalent).
4. A battery operated dermatome.

PREPARATION OF THE WOUND FOR DIAGNOSIS AND/OR TREATMENT

A sterile moist sponge should be placed on the wound, and the remainder of the hand and low forearm should be scrubbed with an available surgical prep solution such as povidone iodine. Pain medication and antibiotics should be administered as indicated. Actual preparation of the wound itself, with the same solution, should not be done until after the appropriate anesthetic (see Ch. 2) has taken effect.

The tourniquet

In treating all wounds, a well-padded (with cast padding) firmly fitted cuff should be placed on the upper arm (Fig.

4). This arm tourniquet provides a bloodless field, permitting safe identification of injured structures while protecting uninjured parts. It is reasonably comfortable for 15 to 20 minutes in a conscious patient without a total upper extremity block. Digital tourniquets should be used with caution in order not to produce local neurovascular trauma or be inadvertently left in place. The availability of a sterile wrist tourniquet is an excellent alternative. When combined with a wrist block, this tourniquet can be safely used for procedures anticipated to last up to 1 hour. If a commercial tourniquet is not available a blood pressure cuff may be used provided it is externally wrapped with several layers of cast padding to prevent its uncoiling and provided that the tube or tubes are clamped to prevent loss of pressure. The tourniquet is inflated after a 1-minute upper extremity exsanguination by gravity (have the patient hold the hand up over his head) and after the anesthetic has been injected to avoid needless prolongation of tourniquet time. The pressure of the tourniquet should be about 100 to 150 mmHg above systolic pressure.

The next step is to do a rapid, thorough, careful exploration of the wound using the irrigating solution. If the wound is too small to permit adequate exploration, carefully make an appropriate extending incision. It is most helpful to use magnifying loupes to assist in identification of structures. At this point a decision must be made to proceed with definitive repair or to transfer the patient to the operating room.

If the decision is made to admit the patient to the hospital for repair of the injury in the operating room, the wound may be closed loosely and occlusive dressings applied prior to cuff deflation. If the decision is made to

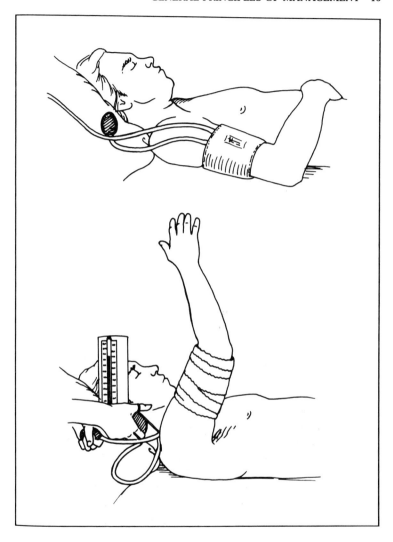

Figure 4
Diagram of the tourniquet set up

repair the wound in the emergency room, the reader is referred to subsequent sections which discuss specific injuries. When the exploration and/or repair is completed the skin closure should always be done with care to evert the skin edges and avoid a delay in wound healing (Figs. 5A-5C). Four or five zero, monofilament nylon suture material with a fine atraumatic needle should be used. For small children it is permissible to use absorbable sutures to prevent the later trauma of suture removal.

At times it may be best to delay definitive repair of deep structures. This is particularly true if there has been severe contamination or if the appropriate consultant is not available. If the wound is sharp and clean, it should be closed and dressed. If contaminated it should be left open and suitably dressed and antibiotics started. Even if the consultant cannot immediately see the patient, a phone consultation may be most useful.

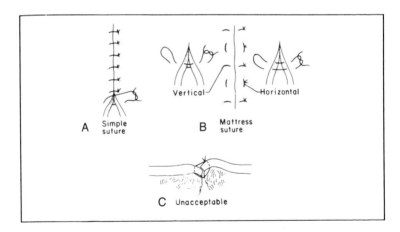

Figure 5
(A) Simple suture *(B)* Mattress suture *(C)* Inverting (unacceptable suture)

MEDICATION

Determine if the patient is current on tetanus immunization. The schedule recommended by the U.S. Public Health Service is shown in Table 1.

Not all hand injuries require antibiotics. However, if there is gross wound contamination (especially with extensive soft tissue involvement), if there is bone or joint exposed, or if there has been a penetrating wound, antibiotics should be given. Antibiotics should be started in the emergency room parenterally. Prescriptions may remain in the patient's pocket or purse while the wound goes on to suppuration. Once started, a 5 to 7 day course should be given (see Ch. 5, Infections).

Analgesics should be given with discretion. There are few hand wounds that require more than 0.5 to 1 grain of codeine.

Table 1. Tetanus Immunization Schedule Recommended by the U.S. Public Health Service

Tetanus Immunization History (Doses)	Clean Minor Wounds		All Other Wounds	
	TOXOID	TIG	TOXOID	TIG
Uncertain	Yes	No	Yes	Yes
0–1	Yes	No	Yes	Yes
2	Yes	No	Yes	No[a]
3 or more	No[b]	No	No[c]	No

[a]Unless wound more than 24 hours old
[b]Unless more than 10 years since last toxoid dose
[c]Unless more than 5 years since last toxoid dose
Toxoid = Tetanus toxoid
TIG = Tetanus immune globulin (human)

RECORDS AND INSTRUCTIONS

The medical record should be concise and accurate. Since the hand lends itself to diagrammatic records, a small sketch is useful.

The patient should be informed about the problem in careful, clear terms. Potential problems following treatment such as infections, blood staining of surgical dressings, etc. should be discussed in detail with the patient. Clear instructions should be provided as to when and how to contact the treating physician should these problems present. The patient should be made fully aware of his responsibility for taking medications, keeping follow-up appointments, and caring for his hand. Paramount in caring for the injured hand is to keep it quiet and keep it elevated until the treating physician gives instructions to start exercises.

Finally, the treating physician must make sure that all the proper forms are filled out, particularly if the patient has a workers' compensation injury. This will aid the patient in keeping his job and getting his compensation payments. As with all types of injury, clear and open communication between doctor and patient, doctor and doctor, and doctor and industry will help provide the patient with optimal care.

2

ANESTHESIA

GENERAL PRINCIPLES

Achieving effective anesthesia in a relatively painless and expeditious manner is critical in the primary care of hand problems. When the patient's pain is relieved, the physician can work in the unhurried and meticulous manner required for the diagnosis and repair of hand injuries.

The anesthetic techniques described in this chapter are useful for examination under anesthesia to diagnose tendon injuries, torn ligaments, and other problems and for the treatment of lacerations, fractures, and dislocations. The key to good anesthesia is to know the proper anatomic landmarks well, use a method consistently to become familiar and successful with it, and to be gentle, in this, as in all other procedures in the hand.

Prior to administration of any type of anesthesia, *one should carefully evaluate areas of potential sensory nerve loss for absence or decrease of sensibility*. If the patient, without looking, can recognize two points of a paper clip about 5 mm apart, the nerve probably is not lacerated (Fig. 6). Another clue to an intact versus a lacerated nerve is a moist digit (intact nerve) instead of a dry digit (severed nerve).

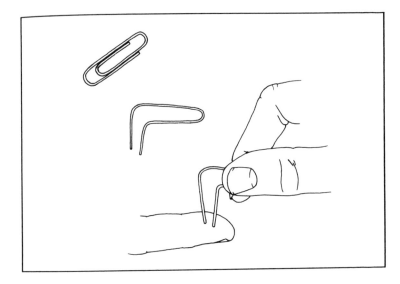

Figure 6
Testing sensibility with a bent paper clip

SELECTION OF ANESTHETIC AGENT

Local anesthetic agents containing epinephrine usually should not be used in the treatment of hand problems. These agents can cause vasoconstriction, which can lead to a loss of tissue if there is precarious end artery circulation of a digit.

Several local anesthetic agents are available. The most commonly used is lidocaine (Xylocaine) in either 1 percent or 2 percent concentration. This is particularly useful for digital blocks. For blocks at wrist level, mepivacaine (Carbocaine) may be used for longer duration of the block.

In any regional anesthetic technique, a delay in onset of complete anesthesia is the rule. One should allow 5 to 15 minutes for the block to "set up." Direct infiltration anesthesia is, of course, much more rapid in both onset and disappearance of the effect, but, if not done carefully, it may add to local tissue damage and may be painful on needle insertion in comparison to a wrist or digital block.

With any block in the wrist or hand, one should use the proper size needle and not inject too large a volume. A 27-gauge needle is the ideal size, using a 0.5-inch length in most instances (no nerve in the hand or wrist is more than 0.5 inch from the skin surface). To cover a wider area, a 1.5-inch needle may occasionally be useful.

In general, regional block anesthesia is preferred because it is less painful to the patient when administered, provides more complete anesthesia, and does not make the injured tissues more edematous. Excellent limited regional anesthesia can be attained with either wrist blocks or digital (base of digit or intermetacarpal) blocks.

With the administration of any local anesthetic agent, it is important to first aspirate before injecting in order to avoid an inadvertent intravascular injection of the anesthetic medication.

Field block

Direct infiltration of a local anesthetic into the wound edges is useful in many dorsal wounds, in certain palmar wounds, and in some elective palmar side procedures. When doing blocks on the dorsum of the hand, use a 1.5-inch needle to facilitate the spread of the agent through one puncture.

Digital block

A digital block may be done from either the palmar approach at the base of the digit or from the dorsal web space (intermetacarpal block). You should avoid a "ring block" at the base of the digit. This is one that tightly compresses the tissues and may compromise vascularity of the digit.

In the palmar approach (Fig. 7), the skin is penetrated at the level of the distal palmar flexion crease at the base of the digit. The needle is pointed first to one side and then to the other and 2 to 3 ml of solution is deposited in each location. To get a complete block, the dorsum of the digit may be infiltrated over the metacarpophalangeal

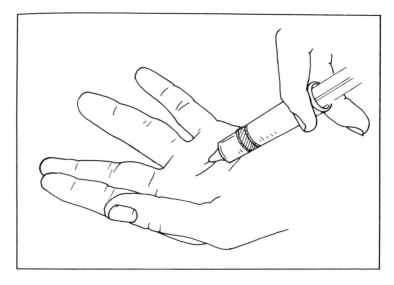

Figure 7
Digital block — palmar approach

(MCP) joint. As with all other regional blocks in the hand and wrist, no effort is made to elicit paresthesias. In fact if a paresthesia is elicited, the needle should be withdrawn and replaced in order not to put the solution into the nerve, but next to it.

In the thumb the two volar digital nerves lie more palmar and closer together than in the other digits. Remember this when doing a block. In addition there is a more significant contribution from the radial sensory nerve in the thumb than in the other digits, and it is usually necessary to do a dorsal block as well to get adequate thumb anesthesia.

The technique of intermetacarpal block is illustrated in Figure 8. The best site for injection is in the interdigital web as shown because it is soft and relatively insensitive. In this area, the digital nerves float in fatty areolar tissue through which the anesthetic agent disperses easily. About 3 to 5 ml of agent are usually required. This, of course, will block adjacent sides of the two digits between which it is placed. This particular block is most useful for injuries to two digits and, especially for injuries to either middle or ring fingers.

Wrist block anesthesia

Successful wrist block anesthesia is easily accomplished if the topographic anatomy outlined in Figures 9 and 10 is kept in mind.

A completely anesthetic hand can be achieved with only four injections (at points A, B, C, and D). At wrist level it is better to use a 2 percent solution of lidocaine (Xylocaine).

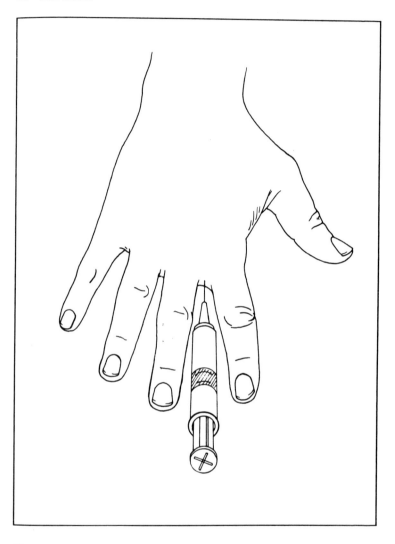

Figure 8
Intermetacarpal block

Injection A—dorsal sensory radial nerve (Fig. 10)

About 5 ml of solution are infiltrated subcutaneously centered over the radial styloid. IV injection should be avoided.

Injection B—median nerve (Fig. 9)

About 5 ml of solution are injected between the *palmaris longus (PL)* and *flexor carpi radialis (FCR)* tendons. The syringe should be held as shown in Figure 10 by its barrel. The operator points the needle 45° dorsally and 45° distally. If it is inserted slowly, the operator can feel it pop through the skin and then through the antebrachial fascia. The needle should enter the skin just about at the wrist flexion crease. While the solution is being injected, the operator should hold counter pressure proximal to the wrist crease to force the solution into the carpal canal. Do not elicit paresthesias. The median nerve lies on the radial side of the carpal tunnel and the needle should point a little toward the ulnar side.

   An alternative site for injecting the median nerve is just ulnar to the PL at the level of the distal wrist flexion crease. This places the needle ulnar to the median nerve and is less likely to inadvertently result in paresthesias.

Injection C—superficial branch of the ulnar nerve (Fig. 10)

Five ml of solution are injected subcutaneously over the ulnar styloid. A large subcutaneous fullness should be created and massaged into the tissues. One might consider blocking the ulnar nerve in the cubital tunnel at the

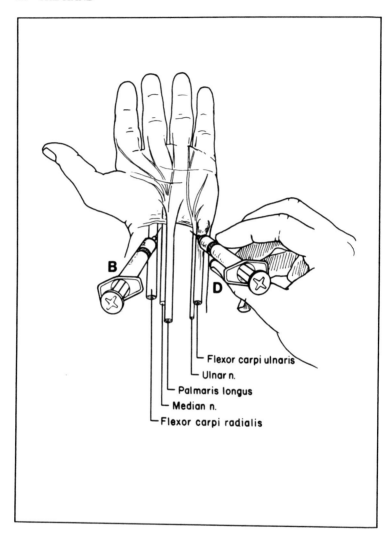

Figure 9
Anterior wrist block approaches

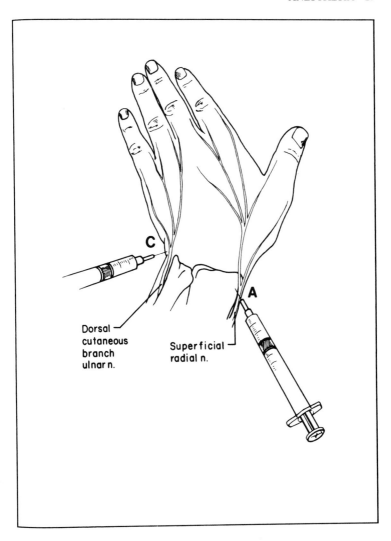

C

A

Dorsal
cutaneous
branch
ulnar n.

Superficial
radial n.

Figure 10
Dorsal wrist block approaches

elbow. However this canal is very tight in most patients. In this region it is easy to lacerate the nerve with a needle and easy to put too much pressure on the nerve with even a small amount of solution. Injection at elbow level is not recommended in most cases.

Injection D—ulnar nerve main branch (Fig. 9)

Five ml of solution are injected just beneath the *flexor carpi ulnaris (FCU)* tendon from either its radial side (as shown) or from the ulnar side. Care should be taken to avoid putting the solution into the ulnar artery.

OTHER UPPER EXTREMITY BLOCKS

Although they are used infrequently in most outpatient settings (except in an ambulatory surgical unit), high regional anesthetic blocks deserve description because they are so widely used in hand surgery.

A block that demands careful attention to detail but that is not technically demanding is the Bier block or IV lidocaine block. Its concept is simple but elegant—the vascular system of the upper extremity is drained of blood and filled with local anesthetic. In execution this demands two pneumatic cuffs placed one above the other (or the use of two cuffs in one unit) on the upper half of the arm. These are applied with suitable padding. As should always be done with a tourniquet, the pressure gauge is checked against a separate test gauge to make sure that the delivered pressure is correct. A #18 or #20 IV catheter is then put into a vein in the band or forearm and secured. The upper extremity is then exsanguinated as completely as possible by elevation and centripetal wrapping with an elastic bandage. The upper tourniquet is now inflated to the usual pressure (100 to 150 mmHg above systolic pressure). An amount of local anesthetic commensurate with the size of the patient (30 to 50 ml) is now introduced via the previously placed IV catheter. Lidocaine in 0.5 percent to 0.75 percent strength may be used. It is important to use lidocaine without preservative. Often lidocaine comes with preservative for local infiltration, but this may have serious adverse effects in some cases when injected into the venous system. Within 5 to 10 minutes a good block is present, and surgery can be started. After about 30 to 45 minutes the patient may complain of tourniquet pain, and at this time the lower cuff is inflated followed by deflation of the upper cuff. Since the lower cuff is in an anesthetized area, another 30 to 45 minutes of anesthesia time is available.

The major complication with this method is sudden loss of tourniquet pressure and flooding of the vascular system with lidocaine early in the procedure before the drug has been fixed in the local tissues. This may cause seizures, and the patient may vomit and aspirate. For this reason most surgeons prefer to have the procedure done by an anesthesiologist, in a patient who has an empty stomach, and in an operating room where resuscitation equipment is at hand. Less serious, are the problems that the field is "wet" with blood and fluid, even following tight wrapping of the exsanguinating bandage; that one cannot let down the tourniquet to control bleeding at the end of the case without rapid loss of anesthesia; that the tourniquet cannot be let down and reinflated; and, that it does not last long enough for some procedures.

Other upper extremity blocks that may be used include axillary blocks and several types of supraclavicular blocks. These demand considerable skill and experience because the anesthetic agent must be placed in the fascial compartment containing the nerves to effect the block. The axillary block has few major complications if one avoids an axillary artery hematoma. In doing the supraclavicular blocks there is risk of pneumothorax although it is low with experienced anesthesiologists. The principal drawback of both these blocks is that sometimes they do not give effective anesthesia and general anesthesia must be used. They are also fairly slow in onset. Postoperatively the patient must support and elevate the extremity until the block has completely worn off. Both of these blocks are best done in the operating room setting with resuscitation equipment and adequately trained ancillary personnel present. This, of course, can be either an inpatient or outpatient facility.

3

DRESSINGS AND SPLINTS

GENERAL PRINCIPLES

Dressing and splinting is a vital part of hand care following injury or surgery. Immobilization is particularly important in the hand to allow normally mobile structures a chance to heal. Because swelling impedes circulation, it is imperative that it be minimized by elevation. First and foremost a hand dressing should be comfortable; it should be durable; it should allow as much freedom of motion of uninjured parts as possible; it should be applied so that it does not slip and slide around; it should keep the hand in the position that is appropriate for the problem; and it should be applied so that removal is not traumatic for patient or doctor. The dressing should be applied with even, gentle pressure, but it should never cause constriction or compression. The swelling that is a consequence of injury, surgery, or disease should be alleviated, not increased.

As a general rule the hand dressing consists of two parts: the inside dressing next to the wound and the outside dressing or splint (cast in some cases), which keeps the hand in the proper position. It is very important to remember that any dressing must be appropriate for the pathologic process involved and tailored to the individual patient's particular needs.

THE INSIDE DRESSING

The first layer should be of one or two thicknesses of one of the commercially available minimally adherent materials (Fig. 11). These may be advertised as nonadherent, but there is invariably some adherence. A petrolatum impregnated gauze is excellent. Several of these gauzes are commercially available in convenient sterile packages. This layer should allow some passage of fluid through it, and therefore one is advised to avoid the use of impermeable types of dressings.

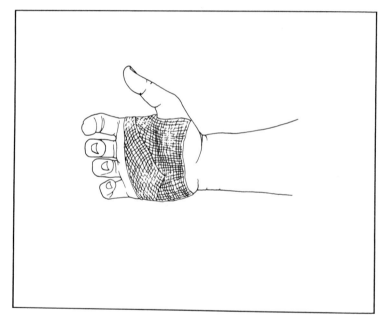

Figure 11
Application of nonadherent gauze

Over this nonadherent layer, place a non-cotton-filled 4x8, 4x4, or 2x2 gauze soaked with sterile saline or Ringer solution. The moisture in the gauze helps make this layer of the dressing "form fitting" and closely conforming to the irregular contour of the hand in the region of the wound. The moisture also encourages the escape of blood and other tissue fluids out of the wound and into the dressing, thereby preventing hematoma and seroma accumulation. A 5-mm thick foam sheet (commercially available) is applied over this to complete the second inner layer. As an alternative second layer, fluff gauze may be applied over the inner layer (Fig. 12). This serves to evenly disperse the gentle compression applied by the third layer. This second layer is easily constructed by using 4x8, 4x4, or 2x2 sponges opened up completely. Some gauze should be placed between the fingers to prevent maceration, but it should not be "packed" between the fingers because digital constriction may occur if this is done.

The third dressing layer (Fig. 13) is a circumferential one of 2- or 3-inch roller gauze, which is commercially available under several different trade names. It is applied with gentle compression over the digits and remainder of the wound area, but care must be taken not to apply this with constriction. In the wrist and forearm areas, particular care must be taken to avoid constriction.

The fourth dressing layer (Fig. 14) is a single layer of some type of cast padding. This is applied to prevent the plaster or fiberglass splint from adhering to the roller gauze (layer three). Of the different types of cast padding available, some are smooth and unyielding while others are "crinkly" and have some elasticity. When treating wounds which are likely to ooze, it is best to use the less firm, more elastic padding. For fiberglass splints, the manufacturers generally recommend yet another type of

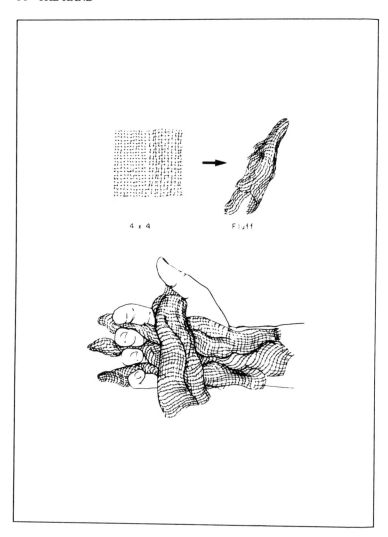

4 x 4

Fluff

Figure 12
Application of fluffs

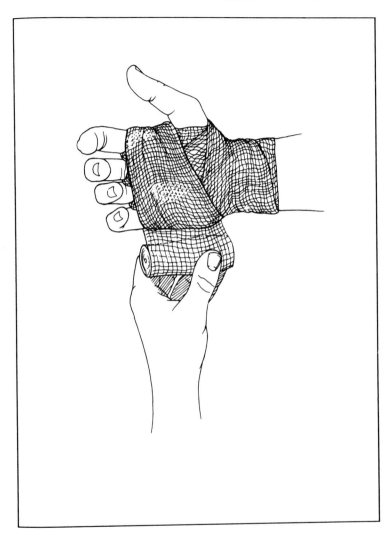

Figure 13
Application of elasticized roller gauze

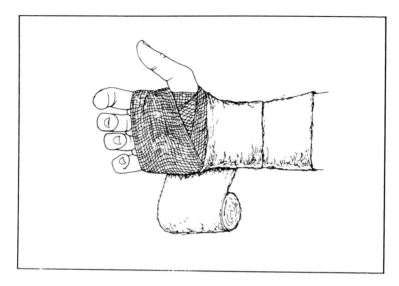

Figure 14
Application of cast padding

cast padding. Familiarize yourself with what is available in your facility and learn how to use it by trying it out on a volunteer.

THE OUTER LAYER (SPLINT OR CAST)

This layer can be constructed either of plaster (more readily available) or one of the new fiberglass materials. Plaster is time honored, easy to use, and, at least on the initial application, cheaper. Fiberglass is much stronger and much more durable than plaster. Because of its durability a fiberglass splint can be used through several dressing changes, whereas a new plaster one usually must be made with each dressing change. This fact tends to negate the initial lower cost of the plaster.

Many physicians use a third alternative — ready-made forearm-wrist-hand splints. However, their only real advantage is ready availability. The patient's arm may not conform to this ready-made splint. They are also much more expensive than splints made from "scratch." It is better to fit the splint to the patient than to fit the patient to the splint.

SPLINT POSITION

Unless a flexor tendon is injured, the position shown in Figure 15 is recommended. This position, known as the intrinsic plus or protected position, facilitates venous drainage and minimizes stiffness. Should stiffness de-

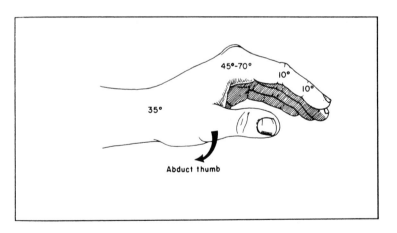

Figure 15
Position of the hand for splinting — the intrinsic plus (protected) position

velop, this is the position that allows the best chance for maximum hand function to be obtained.

The wrist is splinted in about 35° of extension (roughly aligning the long axis of the thumb with that of the forearm). The MCP joints are all flexed, but in an increasing cascade from index to small, beginning with about 45° in the index and ending with about 70° in the small finger. Careful attention is required to prevent these joints from inadvertently assuming a position of extension in the dressing. When splinted in extension, the MCP collateral ligaments contract and permanent loss of flexion of the MCP joints may ensue.

The interphalangeal (IP) joints of the second through fifth digits should be splinted in almost full extension with just enough flexion to be comfortable (10° to 15°). The thumb should be gently abducted away from the palm and, if immobilized, the MCP and IP joints should be in neutral.

APPLICATION OF PLASTER OR FIBERGLASS

As a minimum a volar splint (10 to 15 plaster layers, 5 to 6 of fiberglass) should be applied over the cast padding (Fig. 16). This should have cut-outs for the thenar eminence or other areas that do not have to be included. (This is the advantage of a custom-made splint; it is fitted to the patient, not the patient to it.) If necessary, a dorsal splint may be used to augment the volar one.

A useful technique to make a plaster splint stronger is to make a ridge running longitudinally down the splint by tucking up the plaster. This gives the appearance of a T beam or an I beam. This does not need to be done with fiberglass because it is inherently much stronger.

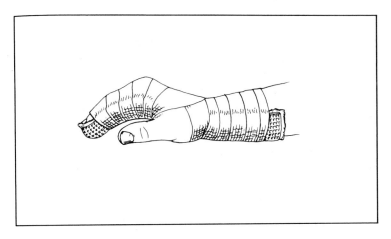

Figure 16
Application of plaster or fiberglass

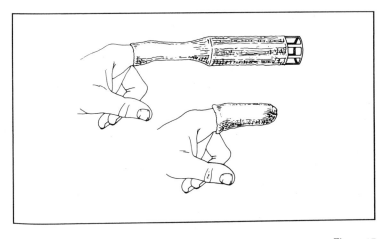

Figure 17
Application of finger dressing with tubed gauze

One should avoid applying the splint material to the skin. The padding material under the splint should extend at least 1 cm beyond the splint material. Cover the splint with a single layer of cast padding to avoid adherence to the circumferential wrap that goes on next to mold the splint and hold it in place. Elastic bandages should be avoided. One of the best things to use as a circumferential wrap is a bias-cut stockinette. During the time the plaster or fiberglass is setting, the physician sets the hand in the desired position.

In general, the use of casts should be avoided in the emergency treatment of hand injuries unless one is very experienced with their application. If there is swelling, circumferential plaster or fiberglass is difficult for the uninitiated to split. The dressing, like all extremity dressings, should be loosened, split, or removed if the patient complains of throbbing pain, numbness, or tightness.

THE FINGER DRESSING

Several different types of tubed rolls of gauze are available commercially and allow a clean dressing to be easily applied to the digit (Fig. 17). Caution should be exercised in applying these coverings to avoid placing too many layers and, especially, to avoid twisting the dressing too tightly after the application of each layer. An alternative finger dressing is to use a roll of elasticized gauze wrapped around the finger and over the end. Either of these are applied over the inner two layers as described above.

Since the digit tip cannot be visualized to check circulation, carefully instruct the patient (or his family) to note any symptoms of tightness such as numbness or

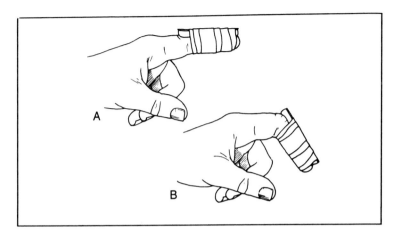

Figure 18 (A&B)
Finger splint for mallet deformity

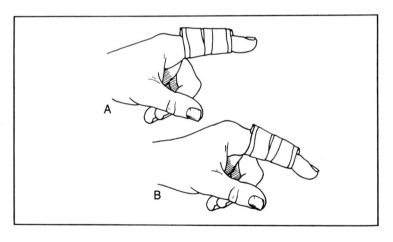

Figure 19 (A&B)
Finger splint for PIP joint problem

throbbing pain. If these occur, the dressing should be immediately removed and the digit inspected.

FINGER SPLINTS

An aluminum or wooden splint lined with foam makes an excellent finger splint (Figs. 18 and 19). These splints are very useful for some finger fractures, for sprains at the IP joints, for some mallet fingers, and for various other problems in the digits. The splint may be applied to either dorsal or palmar surface, but in general the dorsal surface is better because the bones are closer to the surface and better immobilization can be obtained. In addition the use of a dorsal splint leaves the tactile palmar surface free for at least some use. As a general rule these splints should only cross the IP joints. It is difficult to immobilize an MCP joint without immobilizing the wrist.

ELEVATION OF THE INJURED HAND

Patients frequently will not appreciate the value of elevating their hand to decrease pain, promote rapid wound healing, prevent infection, and encourage better circulation by minimizing congestion. Therefore, the physician should stress the importance of elevation clearly and repeatedly. Only rarely will elevation be detrimental (e.g., in the unusual case of arterial in-sufficiency).

The easiest way to encourage elevation is to give the patient a proper sling. It should be designed or placed to hold the hand at heart level (Fig. 20). Because shoulder stiffness may follow prolonged use of a sling, especially in older patients, all persons should be instructed to

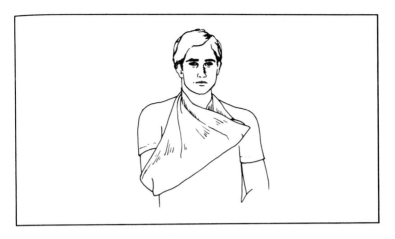

Figure 20
The sling

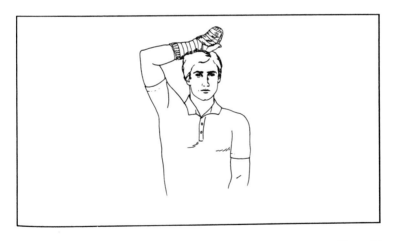

Figure 21
Hand on head

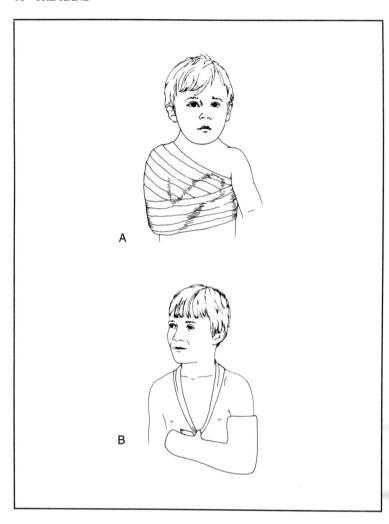

Figure 22
(A) Velpeau dressing in a young child *(B)* Long arm dressing in an older child

remove the sling three or four times a day and actively put the shoulder and elbow through a full ROM. If the patient is too weak to do this himself, a family member should passively do it for him.

With a very cooperative patient there is a method of elevation even better than a sling. This is to have the patient hold the hand on the head (Fig. 21). This approach is especially useful when a lot of swelling is anticipated in such problems as a severe infection, a fracture, or a crush injury.

When the patient is in bed, pillows should be arranged so the hand is higher than the elbow and the elbow higher than the shoulder (see Fig. 50C). Do not suspend the hand with a rope or tape when the patient is in bed. This type of elevation can, paradoxically, increase swelling by acting as a tourniquet. If suspension is desired, the extremity should be suspended from the arm just above the flexed elbow, and it is still a good idea to support the elbow with pillows.

THE CHILD'S HAND DRESSING

As a general rule, the smaller the child, the larger the dressing needed to protect the wound and immobilize the hand. Children will often try to remove a small dressing, and usually they will succeed.

With significant wounds, the Velpeau dressing for children up to 2 or 3 years of age (Fig. 22A) is useful. It prevents the child from wiggling out of the dressing and is remarkably well tolerated by children in this age group.

With older children apply a long arm dressing above the elbow. Care should be taken to apply the dressing all the way to the axilla to prevent rocking on the arm (Fig. 22B).

4

MAJOR INJURIES REQUIRING URGENT TREATMENT

The definitive management of these major hand injuries is best handled by an experienced hand surgeon with adequate resources at his disposal. However, the initial emergency management, even of severe injuries, must be guided by certain principles that should be known to all physicians who accept the responsibility for treatment of emergency situations. These basic principles will be stressed in this section along with some practical information on the emergency treatment of major urgent hand injuries.

While life-threatening hemorrhage from a wound to the upper extremity is rare, it does constitute a true medical emergency. Far more common are injuries that threaten ultimate function or even survival of the injured part. These are also medical emergencies of relative acuteness. For example, limb survival is clearly jeopardized by the acute loss of circulation, as in a near complete amputation. Slower and therefore less obvious is the potential loss that may occur secondary to impending ischemia from unrelieved swelling or from infection that develops in an inadequately debrided, contaminated wound.

Unless associated with severe hemorrhage, major injuries to the upper limb are best managed, at least initially, according to the same priorities established for major trauma anywhere in the body. These are the priorities, listed in order of importance to ultimate function:

1. *Circulation*. Injuries that threaten limb viability are of the highest priority. Unless adequate circulation can be restored and maintained, all subsequent steps are meaningless. Restoration of circulation may involve simple measures done in the emergency room such as reduction of a badly angulated fracture or a dislocated joint. Or it may involve very complex, sophisticated operative microvascular procedures.

2. *Serviceable skin cover*. Providing skin cover may involve simple temporary measures such as a split-thickness skin graft to effect rapid wound healing. Or, it may involve more definitive skin cover via any of several measures including staged pedicle flaps or free transfer of skin by microvascular anastomosis.

3. *Adequately aligned bones and joints*. This priority may be achieved by temporary measures such as external splints applied after reduction of fractures and/or dislocations. Or, it may involve open reduction and internal fixation with wires, screws, plates, or some combination of these.

4. *Adequate joint function*. Both early skillful physician care and careful aftercare by the hand therapist may be involved in achieving this function.

5. *Tendon and nerve function*. In general, digits must have sensibility and mobility to be functional.

Just as treatment follows this set of priorities so does the evaluation of complex injuries follow a systematic format to avoid errors of omission and inappropriate therapy.

Such an examination would include an initial history that provides answers to questions crucial to decision making. Likewise, the physical examination is an exercise in functional anatomy. It is conducted in an orderly manner, and each tissue system is carefully evaluated. The more tissue groups judged irreparably damaged, the less functionally worthy becomes the injured part.

MAJOR LACERATIONS WITH SERIOUS HEMORRHAGE

Lacerations or amputations of the upper limb rarely present with life-threatening hemorrhage. Even a major vessel that is completely transected will usually retract, constrict, and clot. However major vessels will often continue to bleed briskly from partial transections with life-threatening hemorrhage. These partial lacerations are easily diagnosed by the bright red pulsatile bleeding from the wound. A partially lacerated vein may continue to bleed, but because veins are more superficially located and have a lower pressure than arteries, control is usually easier.

Treatment of bleeding vessels should never include blind clamping in a bloody wound. Nerves are often found in close association with vessels and may be injured with this maneuver.

The following methods are used to control bleeding:

1. Direct pressure is the simplest method with the fewest complications and it is successful in many instances. Any semicompressible, preferably, sterile dressing material can be held in place with an elastic bandage. Apply the pressure wrap over the wound just tight enough to control the bleeding while

holding the limb elevated above heart level. If the wound is in the proximal part of the arm it is helpful to wrap a compression bandage around the arm and hand distal to the site of injury. This limits venous engorgement and edema formation in the arm and hand distal to the wound. Typically, strong direct pressure for 10 to 15 minutes will suffice. After that the elastic wrap can be loosened somewhat without initiating new hemorrhage. If bleeding does resume, the wrap can be tightened. However, if bleeding does start again, rapid steps toward definitive operative treatment of the lacerated vessel, are indicated. If wrapped very tightly, the compression dressing itself may act like a tourniquet.

2. Although tourniquets are not usually necessary for control of bleeding, the patient may arrive with one in place. If fashioned at the scene of the accident, it will commonly be narrow and secured very tightly. Such tourniquets should be removed in favor of a pressure dressing as described in (1) above, or else irreversible damage to underlying nerves and vessels may occur. If heavy bleeding persists in spite of a sturdy pressure dressing, an arm tourniquet should be applied. A pneumatic tourniquet is preferred but, if that is not available, a blood pressure cuff may be used. If the blood pressure cuff is used, it must be externally wrapped with cast padding to prevent its unwrapping with the application of pressure. Prior to tourniquet inflation, exsanguinate the arm either by elevation with gravity drainage or by centripetal wrapping with an elastic bandage from distal to proximal. The tourniquet pressure should be about 100 to 150 mmHg above systolic pressure. (If a blood pressure cuff is used, the tube(s) must be clamped to maintain that pressure.) Once

the tourniquet is in place, one should proceed to examine and treat without delay because an arterial tourniquet becomes intolerably painful after about 30 minutes. The limb can withstand lack of arterial inflow for about 90 to 120 minutes, but the conscious patient will not tolerate this. If it is then apparent that operative control of bleeding is necessary, notify the operating room of the urgent need for definitive care so the team can set up. If there is a delay, the tourniquet should be released for 5 minutes once every 30 minutes.

3. If the vessel is far proximal and unreachable by pressure bandage or tourniquet, pinching or digitally compressing the vessel may be necessary to control hemorrhage. In this case notify the operating room that the patient is on the way and they have only minutes to prepare for him. Because of collateral circulation both ends of a vessel may require control.

AMPUTATION OR DEVASCULARIZATION INJURIES WITH POTENTIALLY REPLANTABLE PARTS

The technical advances in microvascular surgery have profoundly altered the management of amputations in the extremities. It is now technically possible to re-attach parts of a digit at almost any level, provided it has been sharply amputated. Realistically, however, re-attachment of an amputated part is not always in the patient's best interest. In many cases, the function and appearance of the hand are better with amputation of part or all of a finger than with replantation. The decision depends on the level and the mechanism of injury and the patient's age and occupation. If replantation is to be performed, however, it is important to minimize the delay. The more proximal the level of amputation, the more important the need for speed. Acceptable ischemia time is inversely related to the volume of muscle in the amputated limb.

Principles of patient selection

These principles of patient selection of re-attachment of amputated parts have been evolving over the past few years. The decision must be made in the context of the patient as a whole rather than by a consideration of just the hand and its amputated parts.

1. *The nature of the injury.* Limb survival and function are best in sharp amputations. Crush and avulsion amputations have a less favorable prognosis for both limb survival and function.
2. *Level of injury.* Functional results vary considerably according to the level of injury. For example, the function of flexor tendons following amputations through the proximal phalanx is usually poor. Flexor tendon function after replantation of a digit at the mid-metacarpal level or of a hand at the wrist level is usually good. (This corresponds to the results of repair following simple flexor lacerations at these two levels.) Functional results of higher amputations, particularly upper arm and shoulder amputations, are very poor, particularly if there has been a brachial plexus avulsion.
3. *Age-related factors.* Children do better than adults.

Indications and contraindications for replantation

Indications

1. Injury to multiple digits which includes the single digit amputations in which the remaining digits are still attached although severely injured.
2. Most amputations of the thumb, particularly if it is proximal to the IP joint.
3. Amputations in children, sometimes even single digits.
4. Clean amputations at hand, wrist, or distal forearm level.

Relative contraindications

1. Amputations due to severe crush or avulsion injuries.
2. Single digit amputations in adults, particularly if severed between the MCP and proximal interphalangeal (PIP) joints. Here, occupation, hobbies, cultural considerations, and informed patient choice play a large role in determining the advisability of replantation.
3. Heavily contaminated amputations.
4. A significant history of smoking.

Absolute contraindications

1. Severe associated medical problems or injuries.
2. Severe multilevel injury of the amputated part.

3. Refusal by a patient to agree to completely abstain from smoking for at least 3 months post-replantation.
4. A psychotic patient who has willfully self-amputated a part.

Any patient strongly requesting re-attachment of an amputated part should be referred to a replantation facility for final decision unless there is an absolute contraindication to the replantation attempt. If the contraindication is only relative, the patient should be so referred. No promise about re-attachment should ever be made, and unrealistic expectations should never be encouraged. It is best to let the replant surgeon tell the patient what he may expect. Patients having a replantation normally follow a long course of hand therapy and rehabilitation (i.e., 6 to 36 months) to achieve even fair function. The patient may require several subsequent operations. Long-term stiffness, lack of good sensibility, and cold intolerance are problems that may follow replantation, particularly in older adults.

Emergency management

Both the injured patient and the amputated part require attention, and it is useful to have two medical persons, one to attend to each of these. Radiographic evaluation should be done on both the injured limb and the amputated part, and these findings, of course, should accompany the patient to the operating room. While the patient and the part are being prepared for transfer, another person should contact the replantation center. For most patients with digital amputations, transportation by private car or ambulance is satisfactory. If the patient must travel a long distance air transportation may be indicated.

The patient

1. After obtaining a history and performing an examination, gently cleanse the wound and irrigate it with sterile normal saline. Dress the stump with nonadherent gauze which is covered by a dry sterile compression dressing.
2. Place an IV line both for patient hydration and for the administration of drugs.
3. Appropriate tetanus prophylaxis (see Ch. 1) is given. The patient should receive antibiotics intravenously. A cephalosporin, a penicillinase resistant penicillin, or erythromycin may be used.
4. All oral intake is forbidden in preparation for anesthesia.
5. Analgesics may be given but not to the extent that the replant surgeon is unable to communicate with the patient.

The amputated part

1. The amputated part is gently cleansed and the wound surface gently irrigated with lactated Ringer solution. The amputated part is not perfused.
2. There must be absolutely no manipulation of the part beyond that outlined in step 1.
3. Wrap the part in gauze moistened with saline or Ringer lactate and place it in a sterile container of appropriate size or in a tied off plastic bag (Fig. 23).

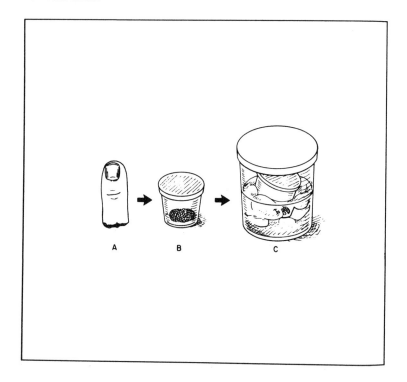

Figure 23
Preparation of an amputated finger for transportation

4. Place the sterile, water-tight container in a large
   clean (but not necessarily sterile) pan containing ice
   and water. This gives a temperature of about 4° C
   which is ideal. Direct icing of an unwrapped part
   will freeze and further injure it.

Incompletely amputated but devascularized parts

Although devascularization is less dramatic than complete amputation, the urgency is just as great. In some ways the initial management may be more difficult. With a devascularized but incompletely amputated part, the wound is gently cleansed and dressed. If the injured part is rotated it should be placed gently into correct alignment and a splint applied to avoid any vessel kinking or torquing. The part should be cooled by placing well-insulated ice water packs around it. Other steps are similar to those described for a complete amputation.

EXTENSIVE MANGLING INJURIES

Mangling injuries usually occur in industry or on the farm and involve equipment such as hydraulic presses, injection molds, routers, milling machines, rolling bars, conveyor belts, and power saws. Incorrect use of home tools such as power lawn mowers and snow blowers may also cause these injuries. The goal of emergency care with such injuries is to salvage all viable and useful tissue. Tissue initially viable may later die because subsequent swelling compromises circulation. Similarly, healing and functional recovery will be delayed if infection develops.

Wound management

Initial wound care

Initial wound care involves adequate debridement of obviously devitalized tissue by removing all foreign bodies and heavily contaminated tissue prior to closure. If the wound can only be closed with tension, it should be left open and closed either with a skin graft or by delayed primary closure.

Delineation of viable and nonviable tissue may be difficult. It is better to err on the side of removing too little rather than too much tissue. These are some guideposts for distinguishing viable and nonviable tissues:

1. Observe freshly cut tissue to see if it bleeds.
2. Look for reactive hyperemia following tourniquet removal.
3. Two ml of 10 percent fluorescein may be injected intravenously. When viewed under a Woods (ultraviolet) lamp in a darkened room, viable tissues will fluoresce.
4. The second-look technique may be used. This is a second operative inspection 2 or 3 days after the initial one when tissue demarcation is usually more definite. This requires a second anesthetic but the procedure is often combined with a skin graft or delayed primary closure.

Prevention of swelling

Initial care must also prevent post-traumatic, postsurgical swelling. This means that tissues must be closed loosely or left open (see above). It also means that investing fascia, particularly in the forearm, should be widely opened and never under any circumstances sutured closed. (See the following section on compartment syndromes.)

Skeletal alignment

Once debridement and irrigation are completed, fractures should be aligned and stabilized by appropriate methods. These methods may include simple external splints, percutaneous placement of K-wires, open reduction and fixation with wires, plates, screws, or a combination of these. Traction is very rarely indicated in hand fractures because of the stress it places on small joints. It is better to use more direct methods of stabilization in the hand.

A final consideration in the treatment of this category of injuries is temporarily saving viable but not functionally useful tissue. For example, a severely damaged index finger may have good skin still attached to the hand that can be used as a turnover pedicle flap to solve a resurfacing problem on one of the hand surfaces. The viable but not immediately usable part can be left attached and at a subsequent operative procedure can either be used or amputated (Fig. 24).

COMPARTMENT SYNDROMES

Some devastating problems are far more subtle in their initial appearance than bleeding open injuries or mangled hands. The magnitude of these injuries may not be evident on the initial examination. Certain of them may result in progressive vascular compromise to deep structures, namely muscles and major nerves. These are the so-called compartment syndromes caused by subfascial pressure. They may result from either closed or open injury. Their end result, if untreated, is Volkmann's

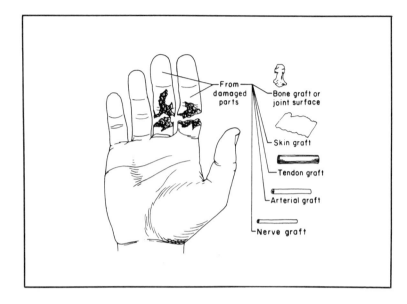

Figure 24
The use of irreparably damaged parts

ischemic contracture of the extremity, a very disabling
problem with loss of sensibility and very limited motor
function. Closed injuries are often seen today in persons
who lie on their extremities for a prolonged period
following a drug overdose, but they may occur after a
brief, severe crush such as from an hydraulic roller. A
tight cast is another common cause of closed compartment syndromes. Open injuries that may result in a
compartment syndrome include stab or puncture
wounds, hemophiliac bleeding, oozing following arterial
puncture, and other similar conditions in which blood
and other tissue fluids get trapped under the fascia and
build up great pressure.

The common mechanism of injury is fluid exudation at the capillary level under a tightly constrained fascia. Proximal arterial spasm may initiate this process but the mechanisms of injury discussed above are more common causes. As the fluid volume increases, venous outflow is shut off before arterial inflow stops, thus increasing the pressure. Finally arterial inflow stops. Paradoxically distal pulses may remain strong while the syndrome develops.

Diagnosis of an impending compartment syndrome is based on a high index of suspicion. This problem must always be considered with any injury to the forearm. The full-blown picture of a tense, painful extremity, with pallor, distal pulselessness, paralysis, and contracture, as described by Volkmann, is rarely seen and then only very late in the progression of the syndrome when muscle and nerve changes may be irreversible. The diagnosis must be made prior to this. Compartment syndromes can occur in either volar or dorsal forearm compartments or in the intrinsic muscle compartments of the hand.

Early in the development of the syndrome, the patient will complain of pain, which is intensified by passive stretch of the involved muscles. Most commonly these are the digital flexors located in the forearm, and passive extension of the digits will cause excruciating pain. However, digital extensor or intrinsic muscles can also be involved in a compartment syndrome, and the muscles suspected of being involved should be tested by passive stretch. As the syndrome progresses, passive stretch of the involved muscles will become more and more difficult and eventually will not be possible. Test the extensors by passive flexion of the wrist and of the digits at the MCP joints. Test the intrinsics by holding the MCP joints in full extension and attempting to passively flex the IP joints.

At the same time the muscles are going through the events described above, the nerves in the involved area undergo compression which is first manifested as intense pain and paresthesias and ultimately by anesthesia.

During this time the peripheral pulses may continue palpable and strong. The forearm is usually not markedly swollen, but it becomes very hard, tense, and tender. The hand when involved is usually very swollen. The hand frozen in the "intrinsic plus" position with an adducted thumb is only seen late.

Physical examination remains the most valuable method of diagnosing compartment syndromes in the upper extremity. The measurement of intracompartmental pressure has come into wider use in recent years and may be used in the upper extremity although it is probably of more value in the lower extremity. Basically this involves placing a needle, catheter, or wick connected to a pressure measuring system into the involved compartment and measuring the pressure (Fig. 25). Pressures over 30 mmHg are considered dangerously high for periods of more than 8 hours, and these patients should have a fasciotomy. Pressures may rise gradually over a period of several hours and, if a compartment syndrome is suspected but pressures are normal, the patient should be observed and repeat measurements performed.

Compartment pressures should be compared with arterial diastolic pressure. Hypotension exacerbates tissue ischemia in compartment syndromes, whereas hypertension provides an increased margin or protection. When in doubt the best course of action is to proceed with compartment decompression.

Treatment of compartment syndromes is surgical, and urgently so. All constricting fascia must be widely opened and left open. This, of course, involves a generous skin

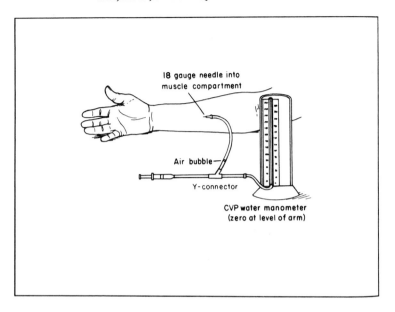

Figure 25
The measurement of subfascial pressure in a suspected compartment syndrome

incision, which also must be left open. Any necrotic muscle is removed. Closure is always secondary and almost always involves a skin graft 3 to 5 days after the fasciotomy. Fasciotomy is a major procedure and usually requires general anesthesia. Certainly IV xylocaine is contraindicated, and most anesthesiologists do not like to do nerve blocks in this situation. In a desperately ill comatose patient the procedure could be done without anesthesia. All involved fascial compartments must be opened. As with any other surgical procedures in the upper extremity, flexion creases should not be incised at a right angle, and iatrogrenic damage to tendons, vessels, and nerves should be assiduously avoided. If the problem of an impending compartment syndrome is recognized and treated early, good function often will be regained. About the only contraindication to surgery is a patient who has a condition in which life would be threatened by anesthesia or blood loss (e.g., a patient therapeutically anticoagulated for pulmonary embolus).

HIGH PRESSURE INJECTION INJURIES

Toxic substances such as plastics, paints, sealants, or lubricants may be accidentally injected, usually into the digits, under pressures that vary from a few hundred to a few thousand pounds per square inch. Commonly a workman reports accidentally discharging the spray gun while using his index finger to wipe the spray nozzle unit. The initial appearance of the wound is deceptively benign with the only visible evidence a pinpoint hole on the finger pad. A few hours after the injury, pain is usually intense and tenderness will be present along the course that the foreign material traveled (Fig. 26).

Radiographs of the soft tissues may define the extent of the injection if the material is radiopaque (e.g., leaded paint). Definitive treatment is exposure and removal of the foreign material under appropriate anesthesia (high regional or general) in an operating room. Propelled by high pressure, the injected substance may dissect far proximally within tendon sheaths and along fascial soft-tissue planes. Debridement may require a finger tip-to-forearm incision although usually the substance will not go beyond the mid-palm. Debridement may be

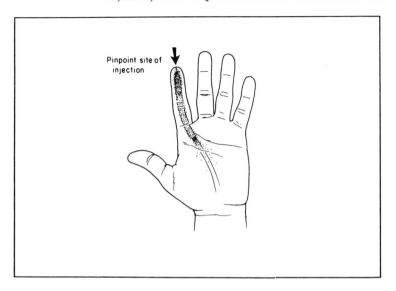

Figure 26
The path of foreign material injected into a finger under high pressure

difficult because of tissue penetration, and the procedure can be very time consuming. It may be necessary to sacrifice some soft tissue, and a "second-look" (see above) may be necessary. Wounds should be left open.

Even with optimal treatment in terms of both promptness and extent, a functionless digit that requires amputation may be the end result. The critical point to remember with both compartment syndromes and injection injuries is that they are deceptively benign appearing at their outset, but both require urgent surgical treatment to give the patient a chance for restoration of normal function. Neither will be recognized unless the problem is known.

5

MAJOR INJURIES REQUIRING
EARLY TREATMENT

BURNS

Included in the general category of "burns" are injuries
due to noxious chemicals, electric currents, and extremes
of cold. In all of these injuries, tissue is destroyed by
nonmechanical force. The most common of these, of
course, are thermal injuries caused by flames, hot objects,
or hot substances. The hand is at great risk of burn injury
because normal use frequently exposes it to these nonmechanical forces.

Thermal injuries

The key to effective treatment of thermal burns is to
determine the depth of injury early. In general, injuries
caused by hot liquids produce partial thickness destruction. Flame burns or those caused by contact with hot
metals may produce deep partial or full thickness tissue
loss.

There is a time honored mnemonic to distinguish
between first, second, and third degree thermal burns.
While not always completely accurate it is useful. It is R,

B, C: red = first degree, blister = second degree, charred = third degree. The real problem comes with second degree burns which can be either barely beyond first degree or almost third degree. The determination of burn depth is discussed in greater detail in the paragraphs that follow.

First degree burns

With a first degree or superficial burn there is erythema and often a few small blisters. Although these burns may be quite painful, they are seldom serious, and basic first aid measures are all that are required. The hand is first rinsed in cool tap water and then gently cleansed with a mild soap solution. The patient can usually do this by himself. The burned areas are then dressed with non-adherent petrolatum based dressings and wrapped with sterile gauze. It is very important that the hand be kept elevated, and the patient should be fitted with a sling. The patient should be re-examined within 2 days. Antibiotics are not necessary with first degree burns.

Second degree burns

With second degree burns the injury involves a partial thickness of the skin (Fig. 27). The resulting complications depend on what percent of the skin's thickness is destroyed. For this reason palmar skin, which is thicker than dorsal skin, can sustain and recover from a deeper burn than can dorsal hand skin. With second degree burns (partial thickness burns) there is deep erythema and extensive blistering. This differs clinically from a first degree burn in the longer healing time required and the greater likelihood of edema, infection, and ultimate scarring. Histologically a cross section of skin will show a deeper injury.

Blisters should be allowed to rupture spontaneously. Before and after rupture they should be protected by a petrolatum based nonadherent gauze dressing and a hand-forearm splint in the intrinsic plus position (see Ch. 3). Many surgeons apply an anti-infective agent such as 1 percent silver sulfadiazine (Silvadene). The patient should be seen in an outpatient facility each day for cleansing of the burn wound and reapplication of silver sulfadiazine and a protective dressing and the splint. Observe the hand for any sign of infection, swelling, or delay in healing. During the dressing changes put the patient's hand through a full ROM. Burn patients benefit from early referral to a hand therapist for education in

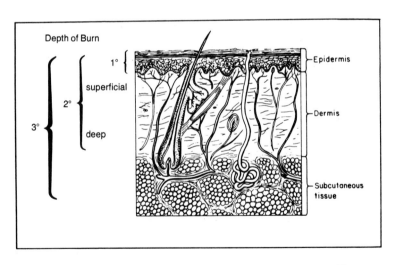

Figure 27
Cross section of skin

ROM exercises. Before motion is lost and joints allowed to contract, the therapist can fabricate removable, re-usable thermoplastic splints to maintain the hand in the "protected position" (see Ch. 8) between sessions of ROM exercises. The therapist may also order pressure garments that are worn in helping to flatten and decrease scarring after healing has taken place.

Healing usually occurs from deep uninjured epithelial elements in 10 to 15 days. Deep partial thickness burns may progress to full thickness loss if infection occurs, and therefore close supervision is essential. On the dorsum of the hand if epithelialization does not occur in 2 weeks, the burn eschar should be excised and the area covered with a thick (16 to 18/1000-inch) split thickness skin graft. Otherwise the burn may heal with so much cicatrix that hand function will be seriously compromised.

Third degree burns

A third degree burn is one in which there is loss of the complete thickness of the skin with destruction of the deep layer of the epithelium (Fig. 27). The skin will appear tight and parchment-like with a color ranging from dirty cream to yellow gray to mahogany. There is no sensibility in this burned skin. The viability of ques-tionably necrotic skin can be tested by giving 2 ml of 10 percent fluorescein intravenously and observing the area for fluorescence under a Woods (ultra-violet) lamp in a darkened room. Patients with a third degree (full thick-ness) burn should be admitted to the hospital for early excision of the burn eschar and application of a skin graft. If the burn is circumferential, it may be necessary to perform an emergency escharotomy to maintain or restore distal circulation. There is little to be gained by a delay in operating if the patient is otherwise in good condition.

A fourth degree burn is one which involves deep vital structures of the digit or hand, such as tendons. Amputation is often advisable, but sometimes useful portions of functionally useless digits can be salvaged for use elsewhere on the hand. An example of this is the "turnover flap" of viable palmar skin used to resurface a burned area on the dorsum.

While most burns are caused by flames, hot substances cause a significant number, and some of these (e.g., tar) form an adherent coating over the burned area. Interestingly enough, cooled tar is not a bad dressing, and one should be careful not to inflict more damage by removal efforts. Tar will slowly dissolve over a day or two if petrolatum jelly or an antibiotic based in petrolatum jelly is applied every 6 to 12 hours.

CHEMICAL BURNS

The cornerstone of the treatment of chemical burns is copious water irrigation: put the hand under a running cold water tap. If the chemical is known to be an alkali, follow this by lavage with dilute acetic acid. With acid burns use dilute sodium bicarbonate. Phenol (carbolic acid) is neutralized by ethyl alcohol. A particularly troublesome chemical burn is caused by hydrofluoric acid (HF). This chemical, often used for etching glass, causes a burn that characteristically burrows and spreads, causing increasingly painful lesions which may not be symptomatic immediately. If the agent is known to be HF, follow the cold water flush by application of benzalkonium chloride (Zephiran) and inject 10 percent calcium gluconate locally through a fine (27-or 30-gauge) needle. Local injection of calcium gluconate within the digit must be done with caution so as not to produce vascular compromise from an excessive volume of injection. In early treatment of superficial HF burns, 10 percent calcium gluconate can also be applied topically by mixing it in sterile KY jelly. Primary or secondary debridement of skin and especially of nails may be necessary before the burn can start to heal.

ELECTRICAL INJURY

It is important to distinguish between a thermal injury caused by an electric flash or spark (a thermal injury) and an electrical injury caused by the passage of electrical current through living tissue. In general, currents less than 500 volts will not cause a true electrical injury. However, a current over 500 volts will traverse through tissue planes of least resistance (blood vessels and nerves) and cause extensive tissue damage remote from the site of entrance. Always look for both the entrance and exit wounds caused by the current. There may also be an "arc" wound where the current jumps from one part of the body to another (frequently the axilla). Patients with an electrical injury should be admitted to the hospital and have a careful systemic evaluation (including ECG). Watch them very closely for evidence of tissue necrosis. With almost every electrical injury there is some tissue necrosis, which will require early debridement and secondary reconstruction.

COLD INJURY

The severity of injuries caused by exposure to cold depends both on the duration of exposure and the temperature involved. The following factors may increase the severity of the injury: (1) wetness, (2) dependency, (3) vasospasm, (4) open wounds, (5) constrictive clothing, and (6) cramped immobile body positions.

Frequently the patient is unaware of the injury while it is occurring. Early symptoms of frostbite are burning and itching with erythema. This complex of symptoms is also known as chilblains. These complaints may be exacerbated during rewarming with development of edema and cyanotic rubor. With frostbite, the damaged hand becomes cold and numb during exposure. During rewarming the patient may experience burning, paresthesias, and aching pain in the hand.

Vesicles are common with all degrees of cold injury and may contain clear or bloody fluid. Ulcers may develop as the vesicles clear. First degree frostbite is a superficial injury with full recovery usually in 10 to 20 days. Second degree frostbite refers to a partial thickness loss of dermis, and the degree of permanent damage will correspond to the depth of the injury. Third degree frostbite is full thickness loss of dermis that will require resurfacing. Fourth degree indicates involvement of deep vital structures such as tendons, bones, and joints and often requires amputation.

In treatment of frostbitten limbs, remove wet, cold, constrictive garments at once and avoid further exposure to cold. Then rewarm the cold injured extremity in water at 40 to 42° C. Carefully dress and splint the injured hand following principles outlined in Chapter 3. The vesicles should be left intact and debrided after they rupture or become dry and hard.

With severe or extensive cold injury the rewarming may be very painful, and analgesics will be required. If the patient is systemically hypothermic and vasoconstricted, core rewarming as well as local rewarming may be required. Antithrombotic therapy (heparin, aspirin, low molecular weight dextran) may be considered. In very severe cases, a temporary sympathectomy by stellate ganglion block may be beneficial. Neither of these measures are highly successful. Patients should be warned that the injured digits or hand will always be more cold sensitive than before injury.

INFECTIONS

Most hand infections are "surgical" rather than "medical" and require incision and drainage and often debridement. Antibiotic therapy is used as an adjunct to the surgery. Hand infections may be divided into those that may be treated in the OPD and those that require admitting the patient to the hospital either for surgical treatment in the operating room, systemic antibiotic therapy, or both.

A careful history, especially regarding the mechanism of injury, is most important. Inquire about prior systemic infections, diabetes, gout, coagulopathies, alcohol or drug abuse, and any allergies. Examination should include inspection of the entire limb for lymphangitis and adenopathy, and monitoring of the vital signs for evidence of shock or elevated temperature. A radiographic evaluation of any hand infection should be considered routine.

Infections that can usually be treated in the OPD include paronychia, felon, infected small wounds, small abscesses, cellulitis, and herpes.

Paronychia

This is a common infection of the periungual tissues (Fig. 28). The infection may spread to the entire eponychial area, to the subungual space, or even to overlap the pad. The causative organism is usually *Staphyloccocus aureus*. An early paronychia which is manifested by cellulitis without evidence of an abscess can be treated by antibiotics and soaks. However, if an abscess is present it should be drained.

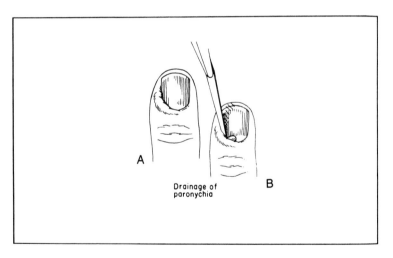

Drainage of
paronychia

Figure 28
(A) Paronycia *(B)* Technique of drainage

Drain the abscess by elevating the nail margin (Fig. 28) after administering a suitable anesthetic (digit or wrist block). Care should be taken to place the anesthetic block well proximal to any infected tissue. If the infection has spread beneath the nail, removal of all or part of the nail plate may be necessary.

The nail plate can be easily removed by inserting a closed, small straight hemostat under its distal end. Then push the hemostat proximally while gently spreading the jaws to detach the nail from its bed. If only one side of the nail margin is involved, only a part of the nail needs to be removed, and this can be done in a similar fashion but with less spreading of the hemostat. Then cut off the loosened part of the nail with sturdy tissue scissors.

The nailbed should be protected with a piece of nonadherent sterile gauze. The wound should have a small pack or rubber drain placed in it (not occlusively) and drainage promoted by application of zinc oxide ointment or soaks. Sterile nonadherent gauze tucked loosely into the wound serves satisfactorily as a wick or drain. Antibiotics should be used if there is cellulitis. Because *S. aureus* is the most common organism, a synthetic penicillin such as cloxacillin or dicloxacillin should be used. If the patient is allergic to penicillin, use erythromycin.

Chronic paronychias are often seen in persons with occupational exposure to water (kitchen personnel, cannery workers, etc.). Appropriate cultures will often reveal fungal infection in addition to pyogenic bacteria. If there is a mechanical problem with some nail ingrowth into the periungual tissues, this should be corrected by elevation of the ingrown portion of the nail or even removal of all or part of the nail as described above. Topical antibiotic or antifungal ointments may be helpful. A recommended antifungal ointment that can be made up is 3 percent iodochlorohydroxyquin (Vioform) in Mycolog ointment (nystatin-neomycin sulfate gramacidin triamcinolone acetonide) in a quantity sufficient to make one ounce. Apply it to the nail bed and periungual tissue four times a day and lightly dress the area. Continue application until the nail has grown out again.

Felons

A felon is a deep infection of the pad of the finger, usually with a history of a puncture wound or some other open injury. *S. aureus* is the usual causative organism. There is intense throbbing pain at the tip of the digit, and the pad is tightly swollen and very tender. The vertical fibrous septae that divide the pulp and hold the skin in place tend to trap and contain the infection.

There are several surgical approaches to this lesion. The most commonly used and most accepted approach is the unilateral longitudinal incision near the nail skin margin (Fig. 29). If the abscess presents in the mid-pad it may be drained as shown in Figure 30. Care should be taken to never cross a flexion crease at right angles.

Gram stain culture and sensitivity of the purulent exudate are mandatory. The wound should be kept open with a small sterile gauze wick or rubber drain. The application of zinc oxide ointment is very useful to help keep the wound open and draining. Apply a bulky dressing and keep the hand elevated postincision and drainage. The patient should be seen on a daily basis until the infection starts to resolve.

As soon as the pus is drained, the patient should be started on a penicillinase resistant penicillin or a ceph-

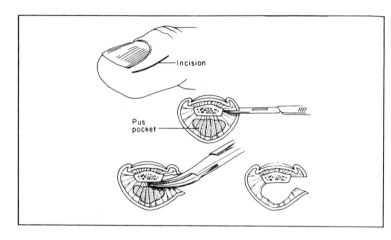

Figure 29
Lateral technique of felon drainage

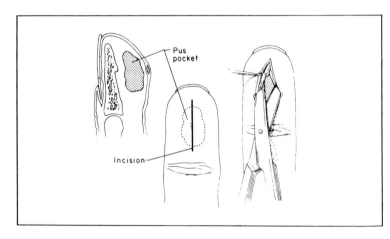

Figure 30
Mid-pad technique of felon drainage

alosporin. If the former are used in a patient who is not allergic to penicillin, cloxacillin or dicloxacillin, 250 to 500 mg every 6 hours are used. If a cephalosporin is selected, use cephalexin, 500 mg every 6 hours. If the patient is highly sensitive to penicillin, erythromycin, 500 mg every 6 hours may be used. An improperly treated felon or paronychia may lead to osteomyelitis of the distal phalanx. If there is a suspicion of this, obtain a radiograph and examine it carefully for any bone involvement. If the bone is involved, perform operative debridement with curettage of the infected bone and institute long-term (4 to 8 weeks) antibiotic therapy.

Abscesses and infected wounds

If there are sutures holding an infected wound closed, they should be removed to allow the release of purulent material. If this is not sufficient the wound may need to be spread open with a sterile clamp, or a further incision may be necessary. With an abscess, an incision should be made over the point of maximal tenderness and fluctuance, and the cavity opened widely. Care must be taken to avoid injury to any vital structures.

Adequate anesthesia is necessary for any spreading or incision. Sometimes it may be possible to place a limited regional block well proximal to any infected or cellulitic tissue, and this is satisfactory. If this is not possible, high regional or general anesthesia is required. In some infections it may not be possible to do an axillary block because of axillary adenopathy. An IV (Bier) block should usually not be used with an infection.

The tissue fluid or purulont material obtained should be sent to the laboratory for Gram staining and plating for culture and sensitivity. It is most important to keep the infected wound or abscess open and draining with a wick, rubber drain, or zinc oxide ointment as described above. Dress the wound and administer antibiotics as outlined for felons.

Cellulitis

Cellulitis is a streptococcal infection manifested by erythema, swelling, and tenderness. There is no abscess formation as manifested by well-localized fluctuance and point tenderness. However, there may be considerable systemic toxicity with prostration and high fever. Ascending lymphangitis and local adenopathy are common. Penicillin will bring about rapid resolution. Vigorous IV antibiotic therapy and systemic support are mandatory if the streptococcal cellulitis cause profound systemic toxicity.

Herpes infections

Herpes infections on the thumb and fingers can be very painful and annoying. They are most commonly seen in persons whose jobs expose their fingers to oral contact (dental personnel and medical personnel in ICUs and CCUs). The usual clinical presentation is a painful vesicle(s) around the pad or nail. The size is variable. Recurrence is common. Definitive diagnosis is made by fluorescent antibody studies of the fluid from a vesicle. This test can be done by most public health departments and some hospital laboratories.

At this time there is no known cure, and treatment is symptomatic. It is recommended that Acyclovir ointment be applied to the vesicles every 3 hours for the first 48 hours following the appearance of the vesicles. This is supplemented by an oral dose of Acyclovir, 200 mg 5 times daily for 5 days. The lesions should be covered with a soft dressing and protected from rupture. Antibiotics are not useful unless a secondary bacterial infection develops. Incision and drainage is contraindicated.

INFECTIONS USUALLY REQUIRING HOSPITALIZATION

Severe infections of the hand are less common today because of early adequate treatment and especially because of the advent and widespread use of antibiotics. Some felons, suppurative flexor tenosynovitis, deep space infections, septic arthritis, massive bacterial infections, massive fungal infections, and mycobacterial infections usually require hospital admission for treatment. It should be remembered that even "simple" infections can become complicated by proximal spread and systemic manifestations. They then fall into the category that calls for the patient to be admitted to the hospital.

Suppurative flexor tenosynovitis

There are tendon sheaths on the dorsal wrist and palmarly from mid-palm to distal middle phalanx. Infections of the flexor tendon sheaths are common. These follow penetrating trauma although that trauma may have seemed quite minor at the time it occurred. The patient complains of a swollen tender finger that is very painful with motion. The four pathognomonic signs of this condition are known as Kanavel's signs: (1) symmetrical swelling along the flexor tendon sheath, (2) tenderness and erythema along the flexor tendon sheath, (3) a semiflexed posture of the involved finger, and (4) severe pain on passive extension of the distal interphalangeal (DIP) joint. The most important and most unique of the four signs is the last. The other three may occur with an infection in the finger but outside the flexor tendon sheath.

Suppurative tenosynovitis requires incision and drainage of the flexor tendon sheath from both its proximal and distal ends. The finger incision may be made either dorsolateral at the level of the middle phalanx or directly on the palmar surface at this level. Enter the sheath between the annular pulleys, insert a small catheter (size # 5 French) and thoroughly irrigate it with either sterile saline or sterile Ringer lactate solution. Fifty thousand units of Bacitracin may be added to 100 ml of irrigating solution. A catheter may be left in place for postoperative irrigation of the tendon sheath. If this is done add a small amount of lidocaine hydrochloride to the irrigating solution before each irrigation. These are done every 4 to 6 hours and Bacitracin solution may be used. Systemic antibiotics should be given before, during, and after surgery. Surgery must be performed in an operating room under high regional or general anesthesia followed by hospitalization for antibiotic administration.

Deep space infections

The mid-palmar and thenar spaces may be the site of abscesses following penetrating trauma. The mid-palmar space is that potential space which lies between the flexor tendons and the metacarpals of the ulnar three digits. The thenar space is that potential space between the flexor tendons of the index finger and the *adductor pollicis (AdP)* muscle. The main symptom with each of these is pain in the affected area. The mid-palmar space abscess presents as a tender swelling toward the ulnar side of the mid-palm and the thenar space abscess as a tender swelling in the thumb web space.

Both conditions require incision and drainage under high regional or general anesthesia. The thenar space is drained via an incision in the dorsal thumb web and the mid-palmar space through a palmar incision between the third and fourth rays. In each case a tourniquet should be used, but the arm is not wrapped with an Esmarch bandage for exsanguination. The blood is drained by gravity. Care should be taken to avoid tendons and the neurovascular bundles. Postoperatively antibiotics should be given.

Septic arthritis

Septic arthritis may occur either secondary to penetrating trauma or by hematogenous spread. The most notorious cause of the direct innoculation is the human bite which is really a human tooth puncture wound. This occurs when the closed fist meets a tooth, and the tooth enters the joint. When the fist is opened, the innoculum is trapped (Fig. 31A and 31B). If untreated, this process may destroy the joint and infect the adjacent bones (usually the metacarpal). A radiograph of the joint should always be obtained prior to instituting therapy.

Optimal initial treatment is surgical exploration of the joint with drainage and debridement of suppurative

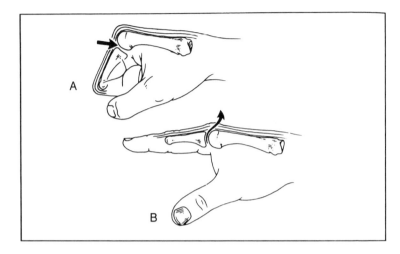

Figure 31
(A) A tooth penetrates the fully flexed MCP joint of a closed fist *(B)* As the digit is extended, the innoculum is trapped because the path of entrance is now closed

material and necrotic tissue. This is done in an operating room under high regional or general anesthesia. The joint fluid obtained should be cultured for both aerobic and anaerobic organisms, and a Gram stain should be done. As with other infections, which are drained, the wound should be left open and kept open with a drain or wick. Although *S. aureus*, penicillin resistant, is the most commonly found organism, there will be a significant number of bacterial cultures growing both gram-positive and gram-negative organisms. It is recommended that the patient receive both a penicillinase resistant analog of penicillin and an aminoglycoside parenterally.

A frequent cause of septic arthritis by hematogenous spread is *Neisseria gonococcus*. It is often associated with urethral discharge. The joint should be aspirated, and the fluid obtained examined by culture and Gram stain even though the smear is often negative. Even if the aspirate is not productive, a presumptive diagnosis merits treatment with penicillin. A prompt resolution of pain may confirm the diagnosis. If the process persists after penicillin administration, other causes have to be vigorously investigated.

Massive bacterial infections

With massive bacterial infections it is immediately apparent that a serious problem exists. Not only is the extremity obviously in trouble, but the patient usually is very sick with fever and sometimes is in shock. Often patients who arrive in an emergency room with a massive infection have some type of incapacity that has resulted in self-neglect, and this can include senility, alcoholism, drug abuse, or some other chronic incapacitating and debilitating disease. Massive bacterial infections may also occur following massive trauma with tissue devitalization, but in that situation the patient is already hospitalized. Clostridia organisms are frequently the cause of these massive infections, but various streptococci and staphylococci as well as gram-negative organisms may be involved. The need for systemic support, culture of the wounds, and immediate admission is apparent. These infections are often life-threatening as well as limb-threatening.

Massive fungal infections

Massive fungal infections are more indolent and less systemically disabling than bacterial infections. However, fungal infections may progress to large, red, ulcerating secondarily contaminated lesions which require admission for diagnosis and surgical control of the process. *Sporotrichosis* is the most common of these.

Mycobacterial infections

Tuberculosis is uncommon today in the United States, but soft tissue infections due to nontuberculous mycobacteria are not. These organisms are found in soil and water and cause nonpyogenic infections that are slow to develop. The patient usually develops a swollen finger about 6 weeks following a puncture wound sustained while working around soil or water. The infection usually presents as a synovitis of a flexor tendon sheath or joint, without much systemic toxicity. Diagnosis is made only by proper culture of the excised synovial tissue or by identification of multinucleated giant cells on histologic examination. Long-term therapy with antituberculous drugs (isoniazid with ethambutol and Rifampin) usually is necessary postoperatively.

FLEXOR TENDON INJURIES

There are 12 extrinsic flexor tendons in the hand and wrist. Three insert at the wrist. They function synergistically with the digital extensor tendons. There are nine flexors of the digits, one for each IP joint. At the mid-palm each of these tendons enters a fibro-osseous tunnel lined by synovium. Both of the two tendons to each of the second through fifth digits enter their sheath together, and in the course of the sheath the *flexor digitorum superficialis (FDS)* splits or decussates and comes to lie deep to the *flexor digitorum profundus (FDP)*. The thumb flexor, the *flexor pollicis longus (FPL)* has a tunnel as well. The amplitude of the tendons in these tunnels is large (up to 5 cm), and rupture or laceration presents the surgeon with a difficult challenge if he is to restore full or near full function.

Wrist flexor tendon injuries are almost always due to laceration. Usually there is concomitant injury of other structures passing through the wrist. Injury to median and/or ulnar nerves, as well as injury to one or both main arteries, presents both acute problems of restoration of vascularity and long-term problems of loss of the two critical nerve functions, sensibility and intrinsic muscle innervation.

Untreated or poorly treated digital flexor tendon injuries generally result in serious disability, although an isolated FDS division may be tolerated fairly well. Even with very good treatment considerable active motion may be lost. Many surgeons classify flexor tendon injuries by location in zones that correspond to anatomic areas of the hand. Any physician who sees and treats patients with flexor tendon injuries should be aware of the implications of these zones (Fig. 32).

The principal aim of the primary care physician is to diagnose these injuries accurately and completely. Virtually all flexor tendon injuries should be repaired in an operating room under regional or general anesthesia. Open flexor tendon injuries in all zones are frequently associated with injuries to nearby nerves.

There is not universal agreement among hand surgeons on the timing of repair of flexor tendon injuries in zones I and II. Some feel that these must be repaired as soon as possible after injury, i.e., within a few hours. Others have

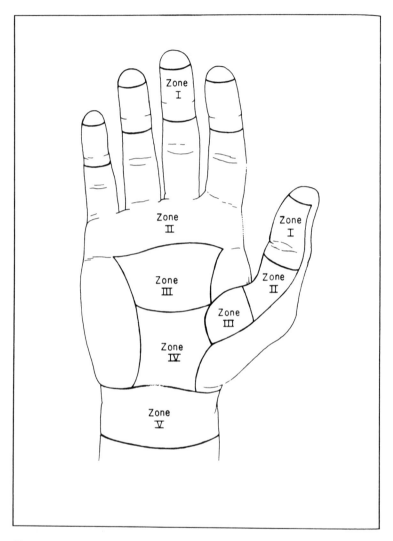

Figure 32
The commonly used classification of flexor tendon zones

found that repair within 1 to 3 weeks of injury does not compromise the ultimate result. This does not change the primary treatment, which is accurate diagnosis and care of the wound by irrigation, closure with sutures, a bulky sterile dressing, and institution of antibiotic therapy.

In zones III, IV, and V the usual accompanying injuries to adjacent structures mandate urgent surgical repair. Initially the wounds should be irrigated, loosely closed, the extremity splinted, and antibiotics given. It is most important that the mechanism of injury be ascertained both to assess the probable level of the tendon laceration and the danger of contamination.

Zone I injuries

In zone I, the FDP has emerged from between and beneath the decussating FDS and travels to its insertion in the distal phalanx. Most injuries are due to lacerations, but traumatic rupture from the phalangeal attachment may occur by sudden forced extension of a tightly flexed finger (as when a football player grasps an opponent's jersey and the opponent pulls forcefully away). Near its insertion is a relatively thick mesenteric structure called a vinculum, which may prevent retraction of the tendon after rupture or division.

If the tendon has retracted into the proximal finger or palm after rupture or laceration, the patient will be unable to move the distal phalanx actively, and the diagnosis can be made by asking him to flex the distal phalanx and observing the level of his ability to do so. If the tendon is still held by the vinculum, some active flexion may be possible. The only way to discern tendon injury in this situation is to look into the wound with the finger blocked and a tourniquet in place on the arm. Repair after rupture is somewhat more urgent than that caused by laceration because the musculotendinous unit undergoes contraction more rapidly in this situation.

Zone II injuries

Almost all tendon separations in zone II are due to lacerations. Because of the difficulty of the surgical approach in this area, it is known as "no man's land." This is where the two flexor tendons enter the fibro-osseous tunnel at mid-palm level. While in the tunnel the tendons change position relative to one another. A very careful clinical assessment should be done on all patients with lacerations in zone II to evaluate the active function of each of the tendons. The examiner should have the patient flex at the DIP joint to assess FDP function and at the PIP joint, while holding the adjacent digits in full extension, to assess FDS function. Remember that viewing an intact tendon through a lacerated sheath does not mean that the tendon is uninjured. The tendon may have been in a different position when the injury occurred and at the time of examination the lacerated part of the tendon has moved proximally or distally and out of view. In addition a careful evaluation should be done of each of the digital nerves because they are frequently lacerated.

Zone III injuries

In zone III the tendons are, by and large, free of a tendon sheath. But they are in close proximity to the superficial transverse vascular arch, the median nerve at its division into its terminal sensory branches, and the median motor nerve to the thenar muscles. While there is often significant injury of nerves and vessels when tendons are lacerated in this area, isolated tendon injury may occur.

Zone IV injuries

Zone IV is the carpal tunnel, and the thick volar carpal ligament makes traumatic injuries to tendons very uncommon in this area. Injuries in zone IV may involve multiple tendons and the median nerve, but penetrating injuries by a sharp object may lacerate only one or two tendons while sparing the other structures in close proximity. Wound exploration of this area in the outpatient setting is almost impossible and the diagnosis must be made by evaluating active tendon function.

Zone V injuries

Zone V injuries are common and may be due to accidental or, often, to self-inflicted knife or glass wounds. Major nerve and vessel injuries are almost always associated with significant flexor tendon injuries. Surgical treatment of these injuries cannot be postponed but must be carried out on an urgent basis. The results of flexor tendon repair at zone V are usually quite good, but the nerve injuries often result in long-term problems.

Thumb injuries

The zones in the thumb are similar to those in the other digits, but there is, of course, only one extrinsic flexor tendon, which often makes surgical repair somewhat simpler. However, in the thumb, zone III is under the thenar muscles, and surgical exposure is much more difficult than it is with zone III in the other digits. It is often necessary to go into the wrist, recover the FPL, and then rethread it down the sheath.

Partial tendon laceration

At any level a tendon may have only a partial laceration. Whether or not this should be repaired or left alone is a matter of some debate. Diagnosis may be difficult. More pain on active motion than anticipated may be a clue. It is important that the injury be recognized and that the patient be warned that a partial laceration can lead to a delayed rupture or a painful and restricting nonsuppurative tenosynovitis with or without a triggering phenomenon if the tendon is not protected by splinting for a period of several weeks. If there is any uncertainty about the diagnosis, the tendon should be explored by someone skilled in hand surgery in an operating room under a high regional or general anesthetic. Many surgeons advocate placing a horizontal mattress suture of 4-0 nylon between tendon ends to close the gap. If a partial laceration is over 30 percent, or if there is uncertainty about a flexor tendon injury, a formal exploration with repair as required should be done.

Flexor tendon repair

The surgeon undertaking flexor tendon repair is faced with several challenges and must be skilled in hand surgery. If the physician first evaluating the patient is not skilled in hand surgery, referral to one who is should be done. In zones I and II retrieval of the retracted tendons may be technically demanding. In zone II the decision whether to repair both FDP and FDS or only the FDP requires considerable experience. At the wrist or in the carpal tunnel, identification of all the tendon ends may be very difficult when six or eight tendons are lacerated. Surgical exposure can be deceptively difficult especially in zone II and with the FPL in zone III.

Results

Good results often follow surgical repair in zones I, III, IV, and V but the functional results are much less certain in zone II. The patient should be told that therapy is usually necessary following a flexor tendon repair, that recovery is a slow tedious process, and that a great deal of hard work on his part is necessary. Postoperatively attention must be paid to protecting the healing tendon while still allowing for some motion to prevent irreversible adhesions. It is not unusual for patients with flexor tendon injuries and repair to eventually require a second operation for lysis of adhesions, if a thorough course of hand therapy does not result in satisfactory motion.

NERVE INJURIES

This section is confined to open and closed nerve trauma in which nerves are partially or totally disrupted. Nerve entrapment syndromes are discussed in Chapter 7. Nerve injuries in the upper limb are very common. As with flexor tendon injuries, the main emphasis in primary care is accurate diagnosis and meticulous wound care to set the stage for early surgical repair by a surgeon skilled in the techniques of nerve repair. The surgical repair should be performed in an operating room under regional or general anesthesia.

Since the accurate assessment of peripheral nerve injuries requires the patient's confidence and attention, it should be performed before any local or limited regional anesthesia is used and prior to direct examination of the wound. Furthermore because adequate assessment of nerve function depends so much on patient cooperation, the examiner should make allowances for circumstances in which patient cooperation may be minimized or difficult (e.g., a child, language barrier, etc). However, every effort should be made to assess the status of nerves that are possibly injured.

Perhaps the most important thing that the examiner can bring to the patient is knowledge of where the important nerves are in the upper extremity and exactly what their function is. Next the examiner must obtain a precise history of the mechanism of injury and be aware of the implications of this history. For example, in knife wounds it is common for every structure in the path of the knife to be divided, while in glass lacerations, structures closer to the surface may be spared while deeper ones are divided. The examiner must also understand that profound loss of nerve function may occur with crush and gunshot wounds, but the nerves themselves may remain intact and will frequently recover with time. However, it may be impossible to distinguish lacerated nerves from nerves that are crushed. In this situation a several day period of careful observation is justified before undertaking surgical exploration. Be aware that a nerve can be severely injured or even totally divided by bone spicules from a fracture.

Following the initial conclusion that a laceration is so situated that a nerve may have been injured, evaluate the sensory area that it serves. Examine for the presence of sweat (nerve intact) or its absence (nerve damaged). If the hand has been soaking, the wrinkles of maceration that occur in normal hands will be absent in the area of sensory nerve deprivation.

Ask the patient to indicate what he feels in the skin area supplied by the nerve in question as compared to a normal area. A variety of objects can be used for this evaluation. Perhaps a bent paper clip with the two ends about 5 to 6 mm apart is most satisfactory (see Ch. 2, Fig. 6). Touch a normal area lightly with the two ends of the paper clip to demonstrate to the patient what is normal. The area in question is then similarly touched. If the patient can appreciate the two points in the cutaneous area supplied by the nerve in question, one can presume that the nerve is intact. Light touch with a wisp of cotton can be used to evaluate sensibility in children and frightened adults.

Since there may be some sensory overlap from adjacent nerves, e.g., from one digital sensory nerve to that on the other half of the digit, sometimes it is very difficult to decide whether or not the nerve is injured. In that case it is best to tell the patient that the nerve may be injured and that a follow-up to make this determination is mandatory.

For the patient with possible mixed motor-sensory nerve injury in the upper extremity, the examiner can add the functional motor tests to the evalution. Once again it may be difficult to get patient cooperation because of pain, emotional distress, or other factors noted above. The major nerves in the upper extremity are the three mixed nerves: radial, median, and ulnar. The important sensory nerves are the 10 volar digital nerves, which are terminal branches of the median and ulnar nerves and the dorsal terminal branches of the radial and ulnar nerves. The detailed examination of these is outlined in *The Hand: Examination and Diagnosis*, 3rd. Ed.

Once the diagnosis has been made of a possible nerve laceration, the first step in primary care is good wound care. The best way to take care of a wound is to irrigate it, to debride the wound edges, and then to suture it, even if it will be reopened in a few days. This primary treatment minimizes the chances of infection, prevents retraction of the wound edges, and sets the stage for subsequent treatment. Proper dressing and a splint are advised to protect the injured area prior to definitive treatment.

Primary or early secondary nerve repair is the treatment of choice for sharp clean nerve lacerations. Most surgeons today favor the use of magnifying loupes or an operating microscope in order to align the nerve properly. This should be done without undue delay (within a week or two), but, unless other structures are injured that require urgent treatment, it need not be done immediately. Undue delay may result in retraction of nerve ends, which may necessitate nerve grafting, a far more complex procedure with generally less favorable results than primary repair.

The patient should be told that immobilization of the injured extremity will be necessary for about 3 weeks postoperatively. Nerve regeneration after repair is never complete, but protective sensibility and some motor reinnervation often can be achieved especially after distal injuries and in children.

BONE AND JOINT INJURIES

History

As with some of the other problems discussed in this section, the most important aspect of primary care of bone and joint injury is accurate diagnosis. This sets the stage for proper treatment leading to rapid, maximal recovery. Often a presumptive diagnosis of fracture or dislocation can be made just by the history. The examiner should inquire about both the direct and indirect forces involved and make an assessment of the magnitude of these forces in relation to the patient's size and apparent strength.

Examination

Abnormal swelling, especially if accompanied by ecchymosis and extreme tenderness, is suggestive of a fracture. Other important signs include an inability to move the joint adjacent to the suspected fracture through a normal full ROM, and on direct examination, one may see and feel instability of a bone or joint or feel crepitus on gentle palpation. A good description of common fractures and dislocations is contained in Chapter 4 of *The Hand: Examination and Diagnosis*, 3rd. Ed.

Radiographic observations

Proper views must be ordered and the physician ordering them must view the films rather than accept a verbal or written report. No one can describe a radiograph with an accuracy sufficient to allow another person to determine whether or not some type of manipulative or operative reduction is necessary. If there is uncertainty, a radiograph of the opposite digit, hand, or wrist can be helpful.

It is wise to take films of the entire bone suspected of injury as well as the joints at each end, in both the anteroposterior and lateral projections. Several other views may need to be obtained to adequately assess the degree of both rotation and angulation. When ordering radiographs of digits be sure to specify isolated laterals. Often a lateral film of the fingers will be returned with all four digits overlapping and be impossible to read with any degree of accuracy. These should not be accepted. All four fingers can be radiographed in the lateral view by using a foam rubber "step ladder" available in most radiology departments (Fig. 33). It is, of course, impossible to get isolated metacarpal views but a 30° pronated

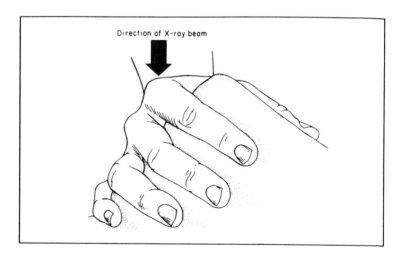

Figure 33
The technique of getting isolated lateral radiographs of second through fifth digits

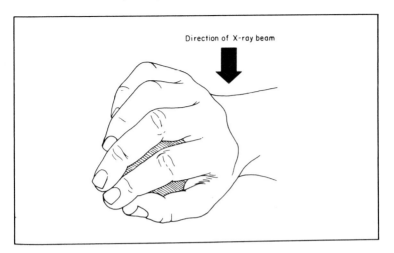

Figure 34
The oblique position of the wrist for a scaphoid view

lateral for metacarpals II and III and a 30° supinated lateral for metacarpals IV and V will give quite a good view. The ordering physician should be persistent in getting views until the fracture is well enough visualized to assess the deviation from normal.

Another very important technique is the stress view. The use of this test demands a great deal of clinical experience and it must be done in such a way that the injury is not made worse. In certain ligamentous injuries, the plane radiograph will look normal but stressing the structure in question will reveal a complete tear. This is most commonly done in "gamekeeper's" thumb* but is

*The name derives from the first description of the problem in Scottish gamekeepers who sustained a chronic attenuation of the ligament from the manner in which they broke rabbits' necks.

equally applicable to other joint-supporting ligaments. The person doing the stress films should wear lead gloves. If the injury is quite painful it may be necessary to infiltrate a small volume of plain xylocaine into the injured ligament or to block the digit to get stress views. Some experienced clinicians use the stress test without utilizing radiography.

Principles of reduction

The general principle of reduction is to exaggerate the deformity and then gently manipulate the fragments back into anatomic alignment. This must be done under an anesthetic suitable for the fracture or dislocation involved. If this does not go smoothly and easily it probably indicates a soft tissue interposition, and attempts should be abandoned in favor of an open reduction. A reduction is satisfactory if the fracture or reduced joint is stable to a very gentle full range of passive motion. If the reduction is not stable and must be held with undue external pressure, it is not satisfactory and an open or closed reduction with internal fixation is necessary.

Wrist injuries

The wrist is an area of particular difficulty in evaluation for many physicians who do not treat injuries in this area routinely. Remember that the scaphoid is the most commonly fractured bone in the wrist, and three or four views including an oblique (Fig. 34) should be taken. Comparison with the opposite normal wrist can be very helpful. If the clinical impression is that of a significant injury despite a "negative" radiographic finding, it is wise to splint the wrist in neutral and the thumb in palmar abduction. The hand should be kept elevated and arrangements made for an early follow-up at which time repeat views and, if necessary, tomograms or radionuclide imaging can be done.

An uncommon and commonly missed serious wrist problem is a dislocation of the lunate. These are of two types: (1) the volar dislocation of the lunate, and (2) the perilunate dislocation with or without a concomitant fracture of the scaphoid. To diagnose either of these, a good lateral radiograph of the wrist is necessary. The lunate articulates proximally with the radius and distally with the capitate. In a lunate dislocation, the bone will lie palmar to its normal articulation with the radius, and, although it may still have contact with the capitate, the alignment with this bone will not be in a straight line. In a perilunate dislocation, the lunoradial articulation is normal, but the adjacent carpal bones are dislocated palmarly or dorsally from the distal lunate. Both of these conditions follow severe trauma, and both require reduction under high regional or general anesthesia. It is not always necessary to do an open reduction although this may be required. Intercarpal instability may result from ligaments torn at the time of dislocation and these ligaments should be repaired.

Another wrist injury that can be difficult to diagnose and can create significant problems is the scapholunate dissociation. This injury results from moderate to severe hyperextension of the wrist. On a normal neutral lateral wrist radiograph, a line drawn through the lunate from the middle of the concave surface to the middle of the convex surface will bisect a line drawn through the long axis of the scaphoid at approximately 45° to 50°. A significant increase in this angle (over 65°) indicates a tear in the scapholunate ligament. Also on the neutral lateral radiograph it should be posssible to draw a straight line through the longitudinal axis of the radius, lunate, and capitate. On the palm up radiograph (especially if taken while the patient makes a fist), a gap of over 4 to 5 mm is seen between scaphoid and lunate, and the scaphoid will appear shortened and have a double density appearance at its distal end (the ring sign). If neglected, the problem may lead to a painful wrist with limitation of motion. Early treatment is reduction and fixation with a K-wire or wires. Late reconstruction may be done by distal scaphoid fusion or ligament reconstruction, but neither of these procedures is entirely satisfactory.

Kienböck's disease is an avascular necrosis of the lunate that may follow trauma or may occur without a known cause. The patient complains of wrist pain, and an anteroposterior radiograph reveals a denser than normal appearance of the lunate with collapse of the bone. Suggested treatments include the following: length equalizing procedures of the radius or ulnar, bone grafting and implantation of a vascular pedicle into the diseased lunate, or intercarpal fusion (STT, scaphocapitate) with or without a lunate resection arthroplasty.

Metacarpal, proximal, and middle phalangeal fractures

Many of the metacarpal, proximal, or middle phalangeal fractures do not require open reduction or even much or any reduction. An undisplaced fracture can be splinted and the hand elevated, with motion to commence in a guarded fashion after a relatively brief period of time (10 to 14 days). These fractures may be immobilized in a palmar digit-hand-forearm splint in the intrinsic plus or protected position (see Chs. 3 and 8) to insure protection. Early guarded motion does not mean unrestricted use but the removal of the splint for a specified time four to six times a day for gentle active motion both in the air and in warm water (see Ch. 8). After about 10 days, stable phalangeal fractures may be put into a digital splint (see Ch. 3) or "buddy taped" (Fig. 35) for another 2 to 3 weeks.

With many displaced metacarpal and phalangeal fractures that are not badly comminuted, closed reduction to a stable position can often be accomplished after suitable digital or wrist block. With phalangeal and metacarpal fractures one should be especially wary of rotational deformities (Fig. 36). Everything may look fine until the digit in question is flexed, and then it is obvious that there is a malrotation. This situation usually requires operative treatment. Angular deformities are usually much more obvious, and it is generally quite apparent that not much deformity is acceptable especially in proximal phalanges and in the central metacarpals. Children with fractures of metacarpals and phalanges can, with growth, correct some anteroposterior angulation, but lateral angulation and rotary deformities must be corrected in both children and adults.

Metacarpal fractures more often occur as a result of a direct blow to the hand, while twisting motions account for a fair number of the phalangeal fractures. A fracture of the fifth metacarpal neck, the so-called boxer's fracture, is very common. The name derives from the mechanism of injury, which is an end on blow to the fifth metacarpal head when the fist is clenched. Because the fifth metacarpal has so much mobility at its carpal articulation, up to 40° of volar angular deformity can still produce acceptable function. However, an attempt should be made to reduce the fracture under ulnar nerve block if the angulation is more than 25° and the patient is within 10 days of injury. The fracture can be immobilized in either an ulnar forearm-wrist-hand-digit splint with the wrist in 30° of extension, the MCP joint in 45° to 60° of flexion, and the IP joints in about 20° of flexion, or in a cast with the same joint positions. About 3 weeks' immobilization is necessary.

If a satisfactory closed reduction cannot be obtained with a metacarpal neck fracture or if rotational malalignment cannot be precisely corrected by this technique, open reduction and internal fixation may be necessary. Angular deformity of second, third, and fourth metacarpal neck fractures is not as well tolerated functionally as a similar fracture in the fifth metacarpal.

Metacarpal shaft fractures similarly may require open reduction and internal fixation if shortening, angulation,

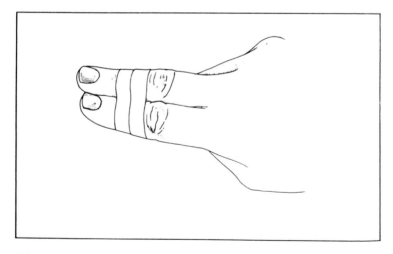

Figure 35
The technique of "buddy taping"

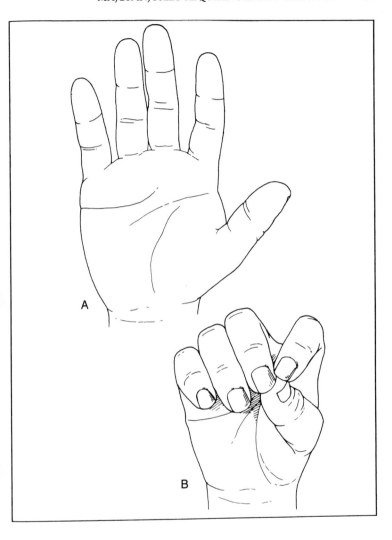

Figure 36
(A) With the finger in extension, a rotational deformity following a proximal phalangeal fracture is not apparent (B) When the digit is flexed, the deformity is quite apparent

and malrotation cannot be corrected by closed means. If a fracture can be reduced closed but the reduction is not stable, a percutaneous K-wire or wires can be placed to hold it reduced while it heals. K-wire fixation is an adjunct to external immobilization, not a substitute for it.

Intra-articular fractures

Intra-articular fractures should be treated with considerable wariness because they may produce stiff joints, and ultimately traumatic arthritis. Small chips of bone about the joint should alert the examiner to the possibility of a significant ligamentous injury. Examination should be done with this in mind. Displaced intra-articular fractures, which represent more than 25 percent of the joint surface, may require open reduction, particularly if the fragments are rotated and cannot be adequately reduced by closed means.

Intra-articular fractures at the metacarpal bases occur most frequently in the first, fourth, and fifth metacarpals. A displaced intra-articular fracture through the base of the thumb metacarpal is called a Bennett's fracture. This fracture is particularly unstable because the *abductor pollicis longus (APL)* tendon tends to pull the metacarpal shaft proximally and radially, causing the thumb to assume an adduction stance. This fracture requires an accurate reduction and stabilization. Often this can be accomplished under fluoroscopic control with fixation by percutaneous introduction of K-wires. In other instances, open reduction and internal fixation are necessary. The Rolando fracture of the base of the thumb metacarpal has a Y to T shaped intra-articular component. Its treatment must be individualized but open reduction and internal fixation is often required.

Intra-articular fractures of the bases of the fourth and fifth metacarpals may be treated by closed techniques if the alignment is satisfactory and the fractures are not associated with unstable dislocations. In the face of instability, percutaneous K-wire fixation or open reduction and internal fixation is necessary.

Intra-articular fractures at the MCP joints are relatively rare compared to the incidence of fractures at the PIP joints and the DIP joints. At the MCP level, care should be taken to ascertain that the important ligamentous structures are not injured. If there is significant distortion of the articular surface, open reduction and internal fixation are required.

Fractures of the base of the middle phalanx are frequently associated with dorsal subluxation or dislocation of the PIP joint. Small chip fractures not associated with dislocation or subluxation can be treated by protective splinting in 20° of flexion for a period of 2 weeks, followed by early active ROM with a dorsal extension block. Large avulsion fractures from the palmar base of the middle phalanx (25 percent or more of the articular surface) may often be associated with instability and dorsal subluxation of the middle phalanx. They usually require open reduction and internal fixation with repair of the volar plate attachment. A variety of techniques has been described including intraosseous wiring, K-wire fixation, volar plate advancement, and external devices that allow immediate motion. Also, a technique of closed reduction with dorsal extension block splinting may be useful. Recognition of this injury is extremely important if late instability or stiffness of the PIP joint is to be prevented. Prompt referral to an experienced surgeon may prevent these latter complications.

At the DIP level, intra-articular fractures of the dorsal base of the distal phalanx may be associated with avulsion of the extensor tendon insertion. If more than one third of the joint surface is involved, if there is subluxation of the distal phalanx palmarly, or if the bony fragment has displaced proximally to a significant degree, open reduction and internal fixation should be done to prevent destructive traumatic arthritis and an extensor lag. Frequently the fragment is rotated in addition to its displacement so that accurate closed reduction is difficult. The techniques of fixation are similar to those described above for the PIP joint.

Digital dislocations

Dislocations of the MCP joint are relatively rare. The most commonly involved digits are the thumb, index, and small fingers. Usually the proximal phalanx dislocates dorsally on the metacarpal head. In certain circumstances there may be soft tissue interposition, which blocks the reduction of the MCP dislocation. The volar plate may become trapped in the joint, or, alternatively, the head of the metacarpal may be trapped by the volar soft tissues, including the flexor tendons, the natatory ligament, and the superficial transverse palmar fascia. MCP dislocations may produce traction injuries to neurovascular structures, and prompt reduction is indicated. It is important to check the patient's neurovascular status in the involved digit prior to reduction. Regional or general anesthesia may be necessary to obtain adequate relaxation to allow reduction. Gentle closed reduction should first be attempted by flexing the wrist and applying longitudinal traction to the involved digit. If the reduction is not easily accomplished, the surgeon should be alerted to the possibility of a complex dislocation caused by soft tissue entrapment. In these circumstances, undue force should not be applied, as open reduction will be necessary. Techniques of open reduction have been described using both palmar and dorsal approaches. The treatment of complex dislocations should be reserved for those surgeons familiar with the anatomic considerations noted above. Care should be taken to spare the neurovascular structures, particularly if the palmar approach is used. MCP joint dislocations are generally quite stable once reduced. Internal fixation is rarely necessary. Temporary immobilization with a plaster splint holding the MCP joint in flexion for a period of 10 to 14 days is generally adequate. Early ROM exercises are initiated at that time. With simple dislocations that can be reduced closed, a similar postreduction program is followed.

Dislocations at the PIP joint are more common than those at the MCP joint. These injuries may be open or closed. Most often the middle phalanx dislocates dorsally upon the proximal phalanx. However, anterior dislocations can occur. PIP dislocations should be reduced promptly under suitable anesthesia, usually intermetacarpal block (see Ch. 2). Gentle longitudinal traction of the finger usually results in reduction. If there is significant resistance to the traction, the possibility of soft tissue interposition should be considered. In these circumstances, open reduction may be necessary. Following reduction, it should be possible to put the joint through a full range of passive motion with no feeling of resistance. A feeling of resistance means that there is soft tissue interposition and an open reduction is necessary. The finger should be splinted with 30° of PIP flexion for about 2 weeks but during that time the patient should actively move the joint at least four times a day for 5 minutes each time. If the joint seems very stable after reduction, the injured digit may be buddy taped to an adjacent digit after 3 or 4 days (Fig. 35). Pain, swelling, and stiffness can persist for months following injury in the PIP joint. The joint must be followed carefully to avoid the gradual development of a flexion contracture.

Dislocations of the DIP joint are quite rare. Longitudinal traction is usually successful in reducing them. Complex dislocations usually are irreducible because of interposition of the volar plate and, open reduction is necessary. Following reduction the integrity of the extensor mechanism and the FDP must be verified. The DIP joint should be splinted in full extension for about 2 weeks after this injury.

Other related problems

Joint dislocations or subluxations can produce disruption of the capsular supporting structures at the MCP or IP level. Chip fractures about joints as seen radiographically, symmetrical swelling about injured joints, or focal tenderness along the course of the collateral ligaments or volar plate should alert the examiner to the possibility of damage to the joint capsule and/or ligaments. Clinical examination in cases of suspected ligamentous damage should include not only gentle palpation but also gentle stress testing of the involved joint. This may require the use of an intermetacarpal block (see Ch. 2). If minimal laxity is demonstrated, protective splinting or buddy taping (see Fig. 35) with institution of early active ROM exercises will allow effective healing while preventing stiffness. If there is gross instability of the collateral ligaments or significant subluxation of the joint, open repair is often necessary.

The MCP joint of the thumb is frequently the site of a torn collateral ligament, usually on the ulnar side. Known as a gamekeeper's thumb, this is a partial or complete tear of the ligaments. It is commonly seen in the United States in skiers who catch their thumb on a ski pole, but may be seen in anyone who falls on the thumb and forcibly abducts it at the MCP joint. A presumptive diagnosis can be made by the history. Radiographs may show nothing abnormal or may reveal an avulsion fracture of the ulnar margin of the proximal phalanx at the articular surface. A stress test can be done by stabilizing the metacarpal of the thumb and attempting to deviate the proximal phalanx in a radial direction. This will produce pain at the site of the injury and may result in a demonstrable subluxation of the joint in a radial direction. Stress testing should be done with the joint in a position of slight flexion (10° to 20°) and in full flexion. The metacarpal condyle blocks the normal lateral motion of the phalanx in full MCP extension. By flexing the thumb slightly at the time the stress is applied, one can demonstrate instability due to ligamentous disruption, and this can be radiographically documented. It is important to test the normal, opposite thumb to determine normal ligamentous tone at this joint. If the laxity on stress testing is 45°, or 15° more than the opposite, normal thumb, surgical exploration of the area should be carried out because the ligament is probably torn off its phalangeal attachment and may be trapped superficial to the adductor tendon making closed reduction and satisfactory healing impossible. Stress testing is of greatest value when pain and guarding are eliminated with the use of a local anesthetic.

In cases where there is tenderness but minimal instability on stress testing, treatment should consist of a thumb spica cast for 4 to 6 weeks. With gross instability, subluxation of over 45°, or displacement of a fracture fragment, operative repair should be done. If an operation is done, the avulsed tendon is re-attached by one of several methods. In late cases it may be necessary to reconstruct the ligament with autologous tendon used as a ligament, by advancement of the adductor tendon, or by joint fusion. Injuries to the radial collateral ligament are much less common. Principles of diagnosis and treatment are similar.

Follow-up care

In treating bone and joint injuries, one should ascertain that the patient has access to prompt reliable follow-up care and that he is alerted that reduced fractures or dislocations may lose position and require further treatment. The patient should be advised that joints become very stiff after these injuries and that both directed and self-therapy are very important for recovery of function after healing.

6

USUALLY LESS SEVERE INJURIES

NAIL AND NAILBED INJURIES

Crush injuries to the fingertips frequently produce damage to the nail and to the underlying nail matrix (Fig. 37). Prompt effective treatment will help preserve both the function and anesthetic appearance of this structure. The most common injury is a subungual hematoma. Characteristically the patient complains of severe throbbing pain. Examination reveals blood beneath the nail.

Treatment entails release of pressure by establishing one or more holes in the nail to allow the blood to drain out. Usually, but not always, an anesthetic block of the digit is necessary. It is a good idea to do a sterile prep of the distal finger particularly if there is a fracture of the distal phalanx because the hematoma probably communicates with the fracture. The nail may be pierced by an unfolded paper clip heated red hot (Fig. 38A), by a battery operated cautery, by a battery operated drill, or by an 18-gauge hypodermic needle. After the holes are drilled, the digit is soaked in warm water or hydrogen peroxide to permit the blood to escape. If multiple holes do not provide adequate decompression of the hematoma, removal of a portion of the nail may be necessary.

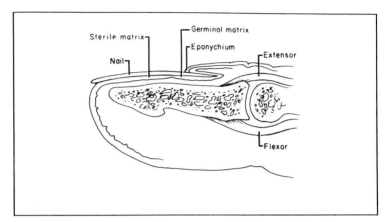

Figure 37
Anatomy of the fingernail

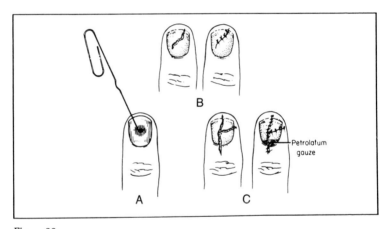

Figure 38
(A) "Heat" puncture of a nail with a red hot paper clip to release a
subungual hematoma *(B)* A simple nailbed laceration repaired with
5-0 absorbable sutures *(C)* A complex nailbed laceration with a small
piece of gauze tucked into the nail sulcus to prevent adhesion of its
two surfaces after repair

When the nail has been avulsed without damage to the nongerminal matrix, the wound is cleansed and dressed with a petrolatum based, nonadherent gauze. A piece of the gauze should be tucked under the eponychium or lunula to prevent adherence of the two surfaces of the germinal matrix. If the germinal matrix (that part of the matrix which is under the skin and from which the nail grows) has not been damaged, regrowth of the nail may be expected over a period of several months.

If any part of the matrix has been torn or lacerated, all of the nail plate fragments should be removed and a careful approximation of the matrix done with 5-0 or 6-0 catgut sutures (Figs. 38B and 38C). A fine plastic atraumatic needle should be selected. It is most helpful if a tourniquet is used, and magnifying loupes will greatly simplify the task (see Ch. 1). If the germinal matrix has been avulsed from its normal position beneath the eponychium, it should be replaced after cleansing and held in place with strips of xeroform. Whenever the eponychium is lacerated, it should be sutured with 5-0 nylon. If the nail has been partly or totally avulsed, it may either be discarded or it may be set back in place to protect the nailbed. Each method has its strong advocates, and either is correct. If there is loss of the nail matrix, the defect may be covered with a small split thickness skin graft harvested and held in place in the same fashion as described for finger pad avulsions below.

FINGER PAD INJURIES

Simple lacerations of the skin of the fingertip are treated by suture with everting 5-0 sutures on a fine atraumatic needle. Nylon is used in adults and catgut or chromic catgut in children. A crushing component to the injury may produce significant hematoma formation in the pulp of the distal phalanx. These wounds can be approximated loosely or left open. Grossly contaminated wounds should be debrided, irrigated, and left open. The patient is treated with systemic antibiotics as previously described.

Tissue loss

When there is loss of pad tissue with intact bone and subcutaneous tissue, provided the wound area is 1 cm square or less, it should be treated with a dressing only and allowed to heal by creeping epithelialization. On the finger pad, scar contracture will give an excellent aesthetic and functional result. In children, even larger

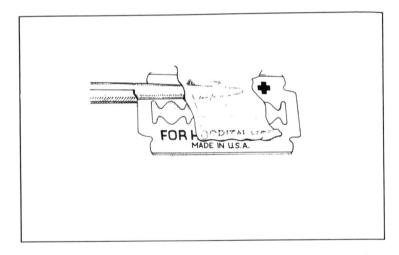

Figure 39
Technique of free hand split thickness skin graft harvest

defects will heal very nicely.

In adults, if the defect is larger than this but with largely intact soft tissue, the wound may be covered with a split thickness skin graft. This can be taken from any convenient area including hypothenar eminence, volar forearm, inner arm, trunk, or lower extremity. An appropriate size area is infiltrated with lidocaine, and the graft can be harvested with a sterile razor blade held in a straight clamp. If tension is put on the skin from which the graft is being taken while the razor blade is gently advanced, an excellent thin graft will be obtained (Fig. 39). The split graft is placed directly onto the defect and covered with crisscrossed strips of xeroform followed by a gentle compression dressing. There is no need to suture the graft in place.

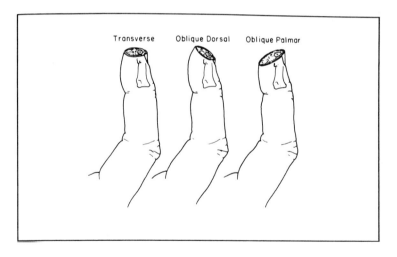

Figure 40
Types of major finger pad loss

Full thickness grafts can be taken from the hypothenar eminence, the lateral groin, the antecubital fossa, the medial arm, or any other convenient site. These must be sutured in place and have a bolus of wet sterile cotton tied over them before the compression dressing.

The advantage of a split graft is that it will allow wound contracture and a better overall result than will a full thickness graft, which does not contract very much. It is most advantageous to use a tourniquet while placing a split thickness graft and to leave it inflated until the dressing is on. The tourniquet prevents bleeding until the compression of the dressing can serve this function. The wound should be examined about 5 to 7 days postgraft application. If there is loss of subcutaneous tissue and bone (see three types of this in Fig. 40), it may still be possible to put on a split thickness graft by the technique described above. Any spicules of bone will have to be rongeured to give a flat smooth surface. In occasional situations it may be advisable to do a local or distant flap. Local flaps are "V-Y" advancement flaps in which a "V" of skin with its subcutaneous tissue is cut and advanced over the wound defect. When doing this make the incision only through the dermis and carefully separate the anchoring septae from the phalanx just enough to allow the flap to advance while still leaving its deep attachment for an adequate blood supply. The flap may be raised from each side of the digit (Kutler flaps) or a single flap may be raised from the palmar pad skin (Atasoy-Kleinert flap). As the V-shaped skin flap is advanced, an incision line is created which resembles a "Y" when sutured. These procedures may be done in an outpatient surgery unit. Dressings and postoperative management are the same as with a skin graft.

Other procedures for fingertip coverage include a thenar pedicle flap or a cross finger pedicle flap. These are exactly as their names indicate. A flap of skin and subcutaneous tissue is raised from the thenar eminence or the adajacent dorsal finger and sutured into the defect. The defect created is closed directly or covered with a split thickness skin graft. The pedicle is left attached for about 12 to 14 days and then divided and subsequently tailored into place. These distant flaps should be done in a major operating room. They will provide bulk, which a full or split thickness graft cannot do. The main contraindications are an unreliable patient or one who has very thick stiff fingers or a contaminated wound. These may always be done as a secondary procedure if coverage is not satisfactory. However, it is interesting and significant that most patients treated with a split thickness graft get a very useful painfree finger with which they are satisfied.

FOREIGN BODIES

Puncture wounds and lacerations may allow the introduction of a foreign body. Under stress of injury, patients may not be able to describe the mechanism of injury. However, they may describe the injury very well and be quite certain that a foreign body entered the wound. Always listen to the patient. The burden of proof is on the physician to prove that there is not a foreign body rather than on the patient to prove that there is one. A radiograph is the crucial diagnostic tool with foreign bodies. Metal and almost all glass will be seen on a plain film, and some organic material will be seen on a xeroradiogram. Abnormal soft tissue contours may suggest the presence of a foreign body.

Any foreign body should be removed with great care under adequate anesthesia and tourniquet control. Meticulous surgical exposure of the foreign body prior to withdrawal is essential. Hasty withdrawal of the foreign body will often cause more damage than the original penetrating injury. Either push a barbed hook out of the wound to prevent the barb from catching as it is withdrawn, or snip the barb off. Otherwise exposure must be such that is can be lifted out of the wound.

Never probe blindly for foreign bodies. Always use a tourniquet and always make an adequate incision. If the wound is clean, it may be closed primarily; if not, leave it open and close it in 2 or 3 days or allow it to heal secondarily.

It is very important to set realistic time limits in looking for foreign bodies. Even if it is radiographically obvious, the foreign body may be hard to find. In an outpatient surgery unit using only digital or wrist block anesthesia, 10 to 15 minutes is a reasonable time to search. Persistence leads to iatrogenic damage. If it cannot be found in 10 to 15 minutes, stop, close the wound, and make arrangements for a more formal exploration in the operating room. Antibiotics should be given after exploration for a foreign body.

BITES, STINGS, AND SCRATCHES

Accurate diagnosis of these injuries to the hand is the key to initiation of proper treatment. One must ascertain how the injury occurred, the time lapse since the injury, and what, if any, treatment has been rendered.

Animal bites

Treatment is similar to that given for human bites (see Ch. 5, Infection). The need for capture and quarantine of the biting animal should be determined by consultation with the local health department. If it is a domestic animal, the threat of rabies is generally considered to be insignificant, but with a wild animal the threat of this dreaded disease may be substantial. If the health department considers rabies treatment necessary, it should be given with the advice and direction of that department.

Wounds should be cultured for aerobic and anaerobic organisms. Radiographs should be obtained to rule out fractures or foreign bodies. A thorough surgical debridement and exposure of all potentially infected spaces should be done. Wounds should be copiously irrigated. Large and/or gaping wounds should be loosely approximated with rubber drains placed to allow for egress of any serum or purulent material that may accumulate. Smaller wounds are best left open to heal by second intention. If a large wound is so dirty or ragged that closure is not advisable or possible, it may be necessary to do a delayed primary closure or to close it with a skin graft a few days after injury. The hand should be dressed and splinted in the protected position (see Chs. 3 and 8). Dressings should be changed at 24 hours.

Antibiotics should be started immediately with either 500 mg of an oral cephalosporin every 6 hours or 500 mg of an oral penicillin agent every 6 hours. If there is a great deal of crush injury with devitalized tissue, hospital admission is required for debridement under general or high regional anesthesia and administration of IV antibiotics.

Cat scratches

These apparently innocuous wounds may result in local redness, tenderness, and local lymphadenopathy about 10 days after the injury. Systemic signs include headache, malaise, chills, and fever. Generally there is no leukocytosis. Cat scratch fever is thought to be caused by a virus and is a self-limited problem requiring no specific therapy. Cat bites are treated in the same fashion as dog bites.

Spider bites

A bite by the brown recluse spider is the most harmful one. These spiders are endemic in the central and southeastern United States. They are usually found in piles of rocks or wood but may get indoors and into clothing. The spider has a large leg-to-body ratio and a rather flat body. It has a fiddle shaped mark on its cephalothorax, which is species specific.

The patient may be bitten while moving logs or rocks or when putting on seldom worn clothing. The bite causes only a slight sting, and the fact that a spider inflicted it may or may not be appreciated. Initially there is a little itching. After about 6 to 8 hours, the bite site becomes erythematous and tender, and a small clear bleb appears. About 36 hours postinjury a faint macular rash may be seen over the entire body. Fortunately loxoscelism, the severe systemic reaction to these bites, is rarely seen but it is more common in children. Its manifestations include nausea, malaise, fever, hemolysis, thrombocytopenia, and a gangrenous slough at the site of the bite.

Immediate treatment of spider bites includes incision and suction of the wound. Total excision of the bite site with closure of the wound may be required and is said to be uniformly successful. If a large area of cutaneous necrosis develops, debridement with secondary surfacing with a split thickness skin graft may be necessary.

Snake bites

The majority of poisonous snake bites are from those of the family Viperidae (rattlesnakes, water moccasins, and copperheads). Snake bites may cause tissue necrosis by direct cellular destruction or by vascular injury about the site of envenomation. Systemic problems may include coagulopathies and/or neurotoxic reactions.

The immediate clinical manifestations include (1) fang marks, (2) pain, (3) rapid swelling, (4) ecchymosis, and (5) paresthesia or hypesthesia. Delayed manifestations include (1) hemorrhagic transudate, (2) petechiae, (3) cyanosis, (4) bullae, (5) necrosis and tissue slough, and (6) hemorrhagic diathesis.

Before starting treatment for a viper bite, one should make sure that it is a viper bite. If the bite is from a viper, there will be fang marks and within an hour of the injury there will be local edema, ecchymosis, pain, and tenderness. If these manifestations are not present, the bite is unlikely to have been from a viper, but if there is any doubt the patient should be observed for 24 hours.

If envenomation has occurred, as manifested by the signs listed above and from the history, prompt treatment should be instituted. Prior to arrival at a hospital for definitive treatment, the injured limb should be immobilized and a light lymphatic tourniquet should be applied just proximal to the site of envenomation. Pressure generated by the tourniquet should be comparable to that of a watchband. Ice packs should be placed against the injured part, off and on at 2-minute intervals. The aim is to cool the tissue, not to freeze it. Unless cup suction can be applied to the wound within 15 minutes of injury, this technique is of little value. Tissue binding of the venom occurs rapidly.

Upon arrival at the hospital the patient is first treated for shock (if present). Fluid replacement should be vigorous to correct the hypovolemia of third space loss. An evaluation of the wound and of the central nervous system is done at once. If the patient is disoriented or shows other signs of central nervous system involvement, the possibility of a severe systemic intoxication should be considered. If this does occur, antivenin is the essential treatment. The patient is first tested for horse serum sensitivity, and if this is present desensitization will have to be done.

The polyvalent pit viper antiserum should be administered intravenously. The dose given will depend on the brand and strength available, and instructions contained with the antiserum should be closely followed. A coagulation profile should be obtained to rule out systemic bleeding problems. It may be necessary to give blood or blood fractions to replace various clotting factors. The use of systemic steroids in treating these injuries has both pro and con advocates.

There are two indications for fasciotomy: (1) envenomation into a subfascial muscle mass and (2) treatment of an impending or established compartment syndrome (see Ch. 4).

Tissue damage at the site of a bite may occur almost instantaneously. Prompt removal of the venom will reduce the possibility of delayed systemic intoxications and further local tissue damage. As with any other wound it is necessary to adequately debride devitalized tissue. As with other potentially infected wounds, antibiotics should be given early.

Definitive surgical treatment is recommended for bites that are accompanied by ecchymosis. Incision of the skin with excision of all hemorrhagic tissues with a 5-mm margin is advisable. Vital structures such as tendons, nerves, and vessels should be preserved. The wound can be closed if all tissues appear well vascularized, but if there is any question of viability, the wound is left open. After 4 or 5 days, the wound is inspected under anesthesia and closed by delayed primary suturing or skin grafting.

EXTENSOR TENDON INJURIES

Due to their superficial location, extensor tendons may be injured either by lacerations on the dorsum of the hand and fingers or by closed trauma to the fingers. The nature of the disability depends on the level of the injury.

The most distal injury is at the DIP joint and is called a mallet deformity. It may be due to fracture (see Ch. 5), to tendon disruption from its insertion, or to laceration. Mallet fingers due to tendon disruption are best treated by splinting the joint in full extension (but not hyper-extension) for 8 weeks (Fig. 41) while leaving the PIP joint free. Use a padded aluminum splint (commercially available) or a tongue blade cut to the proper length and lined by 5-mm thick foam padding (Reston). Although the splint may be placed either on the dorsal or palmar surface of the digit, it is generally more comfortable and more effective on the dorsum.

If the distal tendon is lacerated and both ends can be identified, they should be repaired. The surgery may be done under digital block anesthesia (see Ch. 2) and is greatly facilitated by wound extension. The repair may be

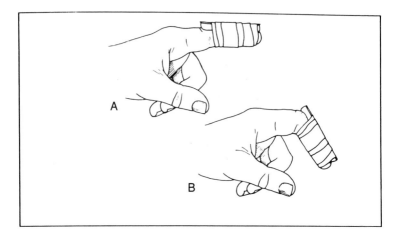

Figure 41 (A&B)
A mallet finger splint

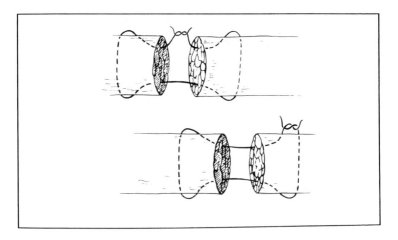

Figure 42
Technique of a horizontal mattress suture

done with a variety of fine suture materials, but 5-0 nylon is recommended. Silk should not be used as it is too reactive. A horizontal mattress suture (Fig. 42) is very useful in this situation. An internal splint in the form of a fine K-wire (0.028 or 0.035 inches) passed across the fully extended DIP joint is better than an external splint on a fresh wound. This is an adjunct to an external splint and does not replace it. It is recommended that this be left in place for 8 weeks. After removal of the wire, an external splint is continued at night for approximately another 4 weeks.

Either a closed or open injury over the PIP joint may result in a boutonnière deformity (see *The Hand: Examination and Diagnosis*, 3rd. Ed.). In the pathophysiology of this lesion, the central extensor mechanism is lacerated or ruptured and the lateral bands, which normally lie dorsal to the axis of rotation and therefore extend the joint, fall volar to this axis and become paradoxical flexors of the PIP joint. This causes the extensor mechanism to shorten and thus hyperextend the distal joint. The early diagnosis of this problem can be somewhat elusive in the closed situation unless the possibility of a boutonnière deformity is considered. Typically the patient presents with the history of having "jammed" the finger, and the area of the joint is swollen. Because of the swelling the diagnosis may not be apparent at once. If the diagnosis is suspected, splint the PIP joint in full extension (Fig. 43) leaving DIP and MCP joints free. If, as the swelling recedes, the patient proves not to have disrupted the extensor mechanism, little has been lost. But if the diagnosis is correct, a very complex and difficult to repair lesion has been avoided. Closed boutonnière injuries will usually respond successfully to closed treatment provided it is instituted early.

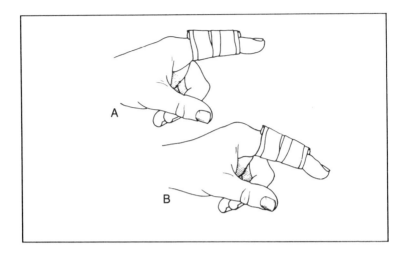

Figure 43 (A&B)
A boutonnière splint

Open injuries causing a boutonnière deformity are easier to diagnose because one can look in the wound and see the tendon ends. The repair technique is a horizontal mattress suture using 4-0 or 5-0 nylon (Fig. 42). The postoperative fixation is with the same type of splint as used for the closed injury. It may be supplemented by a K-wire transfixing the joint to facilitate wound care. In either case the repair should be splinted for about 6 weeks.

Lacerations to the extensor aponeurosis between the MCP and PIP and PIP and DIP joints are usually not complete. At the time of exposure and repair the surgeon can gauge the amount of stress placed on them by flexing MCP, PIP, and DIP joints and judging which of these joints need to be immobilized. In some cases a forearm-hand-digit splint in the intrinsic plus position (see Ch. 3) will be necessary, and in others a digit splint will suffice. In these lacerations a running suture of nylon is very useful. However, if there is no tendon separation on active or passive motion, a splint alone may suffice.

In the digits, retraction of the tendons is not much of a problem, and the ends can be recovered by minimal wound extension. As one moves onto the dorsum of the hand, retraction becomes more of a problem, and recovering the proximal stump, even at the distal metacarpal level, can be quite taxing. If the ends can be found easily, suture material and techniques already described above are satisfactory. If the proximal end cannot be readily found, the wisest course is to close the wound and make arrangements for repair under high regional or general anesthesia in an operating room. Following repair of tendons at hand and wrist level a forearm-hand-digit splint is required. In general the intrinsic plus position previously described is used with perhaps only 30° of MCP flexion. The splint should be utilized for about 3 weeks.

7

OTHER COMMONLY SEEN PROBLEMS

There are a variety of common hand problems that fall into the quasitraumatic or nontraumatic categories. Patients will often present themselves to emergency or general medical outpatient departments with these problems. It is very useful to be able to diagnose the problem, offer simple treatments, and give the patient some idea of more definitive treatments that may be available. Most of these conditions are carefully described in *The Hand: Examination and Diagnosis,* 3rd. Ed. The reader is urged to use the appropriate sections of that volume in conjunction with the treatment described in the following paragraphs.

STRAINS AND SPRAINS OF FINGER JOINTS

Because each of the 14 digital joints has several ligaments to stabilize its axes of motion and to prevent abnormal motion, strains and sprains in the hand are quite common. These are incomplete tears of ligaments, and it is important in making a diagnosis of a strain or a sprain to make certain that there is not a complete tear of a ligament with joint instability or subluxation. The primary treatment of strains and sprains consists of putting the injured part at rest by splinting (see Ch. 3), elevation, and appropriate analgesics. It is often wise to apply an ice bag to the injured part for the first 24 to 48 hours to minimize swelling.

In chronic sprains one may instruct the patient to soak the hand briefly in warm water several times each day while performing gentle ROM exercises (see Ch. 8). Patients with severe chronic sprains may benefit by referral to a hand therapist. Modalities such as ultrasound, gentle passive and active motion exercises, edema control techniques, and intermittent splinting may significantly decrease pain and increase function. At times it is helpful to instill small amounts of a clear steroid into the injured ligament. When giving steroids locally, one must use small volumes and fine needles just as one does in giving local anesthetic blocks (see Ch. 2). There is always some question about whether to give a long-acting cortisone (triamcinolone) or a short-acting one (dexamethasone). The long-acting preparation has the disadvantages of causing skin depigmentation and subcutaneous fat atrophy. In general it is recommended that short-acting, clear steroids be used for this reason.

TRIGGER THUMB AND FINGERS (STENOSING TENOSYNOVITIS)

Triggering can occur anywhere that there is a restraining retinacular system (i.e., in the dorsal wrist compartments or in the flexor tendon sheaths). It occurs most commonly on the flexor surface in the ring and long fingers and in the thumb. Patients with this condition complain of catching, snapping, locking, or jumping of the affected finger or thumb. Although mild pain is often referred to the dorsal PIP or IP joint, the problem invariably is at the proximal portion of the flexor retinacular system, the "A-1 pulley" (Fig. 44). The condition is caused by inflammation of the synovium of the flexor tendon system with a resultant size discrepancy between the tendon and the sheath. At surgery one usually observes both a nodule in the tendon and a thick stenotic sheath. The condition may be associated with rheumatoid arthritis or may follow prior penetrating trauma but usually is "idiopathic."

Examination reveals tenderness over the proximal tendon sheath at the level of the metacarpal head and sometimes a nodule can be felt in the tendon. The examiner can often feel snapping or triggering as the patient actively flexes and extends both IP joints of the digit. Since the condition sometimes is quite painful, the patient will either move the digit with great reluctance or it will actually be fixed in flexion or extension. Characteristically patients will complain that the problem is most pronounced upon awakening and diminishes as they "limber up" the digit.

The most effective nonoperative treatment consists of injection of a clear steroid combined with a local anesthetic. A useful combination is 0.5 ml of the steroid dexamethasone (4 mg/ml) combined with 0.5 ml of 1 percent plain lidocaine. As with many other hand injections a 0.5-inch, 27-gauge needle seems to be the ideal size. The needle is inserted by holding the barrel of the syringe and penetrating through the tendon until the floor of the sheath is reached as evidenced by resistance to further advancement. The needle is then slowly withdrawn while pressure is applied to the syringe plunger. When the needle enters the open sheath, the liquid will readily squirt into the tendon canal (Fig. 45). A squirt feeling is often noted by the patient and may be seen or felt by the examiner. Paradoxically the triggering

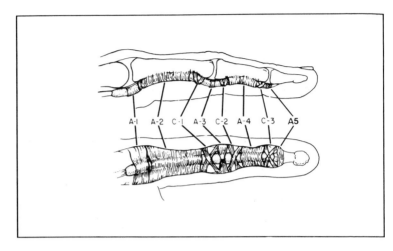

Figure 44
The flexor pulley system in the palm and digits

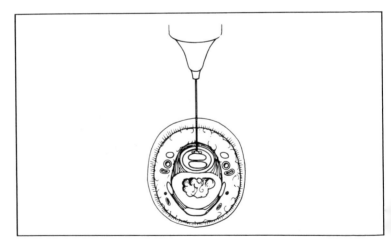

Figure 45
Injection of the flexor tendon sheath for a trigger finger

phenomenon is often more pronounced immediately after the injection, but the pain is gone while the action of the local anesthetic lasts. As with any injection of this sort there may be quite a lot of pain after a few hours and it may last 24 to 36 hours. Some surgeons like to have the patient wear a splint to hold the IP joints in full extension for a week or so after the injection (at least at night).

This injection may be repeated twice at weekly intervals, but if the problem persists after that, operative intervention is advised. The patient should be told that this can be (and should be) done under local anesthesia, but a tourniquet on the arm is required. Surgery is almost always curative. The operation consists of making a skin incision over the involved flexor tendon sheath in the palm, carefully avoiding the digital nerves, and identifying the flexor tendon sheath. The sheath is incised longitudinally for a distance that permits unrestricted, full-active finger motion by the patient to demonstrate that the constricted portion has been opened.

deQUERVAIN'S STENOSING TENOSYNOVITIS

deQuervain's stenosing tenosynovitis affects the first dorsal compartment, which houses the APL and *extensor pollicis brevis (EPB)* tendons on the radial side of the wrist. There may be a "trigger" phenomenon (stenosing tenosynovitis) but this is not common. It is the only commonly encountered tendonitis of the extensor tendons. Typically, patients complain of pain in this area when they use their thumbs. Palpation over the first dorsal compartment reveals thickening and tenderness. Finkelstein's test is performed by having the patient flex the thumb and grasp it with the other fingers while actively putting the wrist into ulnar deviation. Sharp pain noted at the radial styloid usually confirms the diagnosis. Patients will also complain of pain on forced thumb abduction-extension.

Initial treatment is by injection of the first dorsal compartment with a steroid-lidocaine combination using a total volume of about 2 ml. Care should be taken to avoid the radial sensory nerve and its branches and the numerous veins commonly found in this area. In this area a 1.5-inch, 27-gauge needle is useful. The needle is put through the skin at the distal end of the first dorsal compartment and then slowly advanced into the compartment while injecting the solution. Often the fluid can be seen to "pop" through the compartment and appear on its proximal margin. Many surgeons find it useful to make the patient a removable plaster or fiberglass splint that immobilizes the wrist and thumb. This can be held on either by elastic bandage or self-adhering straps.

If two to three injections over a 3 to 5 week period fail to give relief, strong consideration should be given to surgically releasing the stenotic tendon sheath (or sheaths since there is often more than one). This is also a procedure that can be done under local anesthesia with an arm tourniquet. The operation is done through a short transverse incision and taking great care to identify and not injure the radial sensory nerve. The tendon sheath is identified and incised longitudinally. Care must be taken to open each of the subcompartments since there may be three or four. One can confirm that each tendon slip is free by having the patient flex and extend the thumb MCP joint for the EPB and by ulnarly and radially deviating the wrist for the APL.

An important differential diagnosis is arthritis of the thumb basal joint (the first carpometacarpal (CMC) joint or the metacarpal trapezial joint). The distinction is made by accurately localizing the pain and tenderness in either one area or the other. Basal joint arthritis pain is elicited or aggravated by the examiner grinding the first metacarpal on the trapezium ("mortar and pestle test"). This maneuver will not cause pain in deQuervain's disease.

GANGLION CYST

Ganglion cyst is the most common soft tissue tumor of the hand. It may be formed from modified synovial cells. The cyst can usually be demonstrated to connect with the underlying joint or tendon sheath. Usually it occurs when there is a small tear in overlying ligaments allowing the synovial tissue to herniate out of its normal position. If the small ligamentous tear then heals or is pulled together, the fluid secreted by the synovial tissue has no egress into joint or tendon sheath and bulges out under the skin. Sometimes the ganglion drains internally, and this accounts for the clinical finding of waxing and waning of ganglions. Because the cyst fluid may be under considerable pressure, ganglions can be rock hard, but they transilluminate, which distinguishes them from solid tumors.

Ganglions usually occur in one of four locations on the hand: (1) on the dorsoradial wrist arising from the area of the scapholunatecapitate articulation (2) on the volar radial wrist in close approximation to the radial artery and FCR tendon, usually arising from one of the scaphoid articulations but sometimes arising from the basal joint of the thumb or the FCR tendon sheath, (3) over a flexor tendon sheath in the distal palm and arising from the flexor tendon sheath at the area between the A-1 and A-2 pulleys, and (4) from the DIP joint dorsally, the mucous cyst (usually associated with DIP joint osteoarthritis).

On the dorsal wrist the most common differential diagnosis is dorsal synovitis from the extensor retinaculum area. Synovitis is invariably softer than a ganglion and does not transilluminate so readily. The volar ganglion is sometimes confused with a radial artery aneurysm. Traumatic pseudoaneurysms may occur in this area, but one should be able to elicit a history of penetrating trauma. Arteriosclerotic aneurysms are extremely rare. The ganglion at the base of the finger feels like a BB or tiny marble.

Primary treatment usually consists of making the diagnosis and reassuring the patient that it is not an ominous lesion. If it is very large or troublesome, the dorsal ganglion cyst can be aspirated, but the patient should be warned that only the fluid is being removed, that the cyst probably will fill up again. If an aspiration is done one must use a needle large enough (usually a 18-gauge) to draw out the viscous, usually clear fluid. Volar carpal ganglions and midline ganglions of the flexor sheath are more difficult to aspirate and should be done with caution to avoid injury to the surrounding structures.

Definitive treatment is excision in an operating room with care taken to trace the lesion to its origin. A ganglion of the DIP joint (mucous cyst) or a ganglion of the flexor sheath can be removed under digital block or field block anesthesia. When excising a mucous cyst, it is important to debride the underlying joint of any local osteophytes. At the wrist level the ganglion should be excised under high regional anesthesia. An incision is made over the lesion, which is identified and followed into the joint or tendon sheath from which it arises. A small cuff of joint capsule or tendon sheath is excised and capsule or tendon sheath is left open. Postoperatively the wrist or digit is splinted for 7 to 10 days.

DUPUYTREN'S FASCIITIS AND CONTRACTURE

Although Dupuytren's fasciitis and contracture is a very common problem that develops most frequently in the hands of middle aged persons, it may be seen in persons in their twenties. It is unusual in oriental or black people. It is seven times as common in men as it is in women. There is a tendency for it to run in families. The condition is said to be associated with alcoholism and some systemic degenerative diseases (e.g., diabetes) but this may be more coincidental in this age group than based on cause and effect.

Usually the first thing that a patient notes is a nodule in the palm, and it is often first noticed after trauma to the hand. However, no clear relationship between trauma and Dupuytren's fasciitis and contracture has ever been proven. The condition may stabilize at this level, or it may progress to cause a contracture at an MCP joint, a PIP joint or, rarely, a DIP joint. The process involves the palmar fascia and does not (as is sometimes supposed) involve the flexor tendons at all. The order of finger involvement in terms of most to least common is: ring, small, long, thumb, and index.

The only effective treatment for the problem is surgery. If one very superficial fascial band is present, it may be transected with temporary relief of the contracture. More permanent relief can be obtained by removing the diseased fascia. The patient should be advised that surgery does not cure the disease but removes only the tissue involved in producing the offending contracture. The development of disease in new locations or recurrence at sites of previous surgery can occur. Patients who have a greater likelihood for recurrence or a diathesis for the disease include those with involvement at sites other that the palmar aspect of the hand, those with onset of the disease at an early age, and those with a strong family history of the disease.

FRACTURES OF THE DISTAL PHALANX

Crush injuries of the fingertips are among the most common injuries of the hand. The presence of a subungual hematoma (blood under the nail plate) should suggest the possibility of an underlying fracture of the distal phalanx. Large subungual hematomas are associated with significant injuries to the nailbed worthy of surgical repair. Failure to realign displaced fractures of the distal phalanx and to repair lacerations of the nailbed may lead to permanent deformities of the nail plate.

Large subungual hematomas may require decompression for pain relief. This should be done in a sterile fashion using a nail drill or fine cautery device (see pages 113–115).

NERVE ENTRAPMENT SYNDROMES

Carpal tunnel syndrome

By far the most common nerve entrapment syndrome in the upper limb is the carpal tunnel syndrome. Patients complain of their hand "going to sleep" and they are frequently awakened at night with numbness, pain, and tingling in all or part of the median nerve distribution (pads of thumb, index, long, and radial side of the ring fingers). Pain may be referred to the elbow or shoulder. Activities requiring sustained or repetitive use of the hand frequently initiate these symptoms. The condition is often bilateral. It may be associated with rheumatoid arthritis or follow a Colles fracture, and it sometimes occurs during pregnancy (usually abating after delivery). It is said to be associated with diabetes and thyroid disease. It is definitely associated with certain occupational activities in which prolonged pressure is put on the palmar base of the hand or when this part of the hand is used for banging on objects. However, the largest group of patients who have carpal tunnel syndrome fall into the idiopathic category, and the nerve symptoms are probably due to a mild nonspecific flexor tenosynovitis.

Examination usually reveals a hand that is normal in appearance but thenar atrophy may be present in cases of long duration. It is the *abductor pollicis brevis (APB)* muscle which atrophies. If this atrophy is severe, the thumb cannot be pronated (Fig. 46). Tinel's sign (tingling or

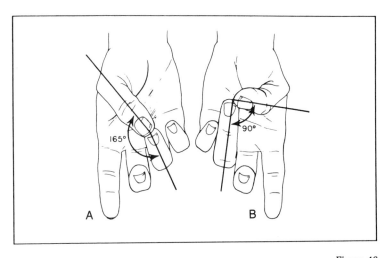

Figure 46
(A) With an intact median nerve, the thumb can be pronated lining up the nails at or near 180° *(B)* With a median palsy, the thumb cannot be pronated and the nail is less than 100°

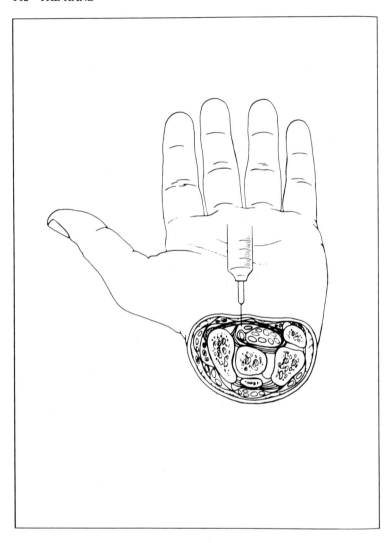

Figure 47
Cross section of the carpal tunnel with an injecting needle in place

electric shock sensation) may be elicited when the median nerve is tapped at the wrist. The most useful clinical test is the wrist flexion or Phalen's test in which the wrist is held in flexion for 60 seconds. This wrist flexion should not be forced. Numbness or paresthesias elicited during this time in the median nerve distribution confirms the diagnosis.

Differential diagnoses include cervical radiculitis, thoracic outlet syndrome, and the various peripheral neuropathies. Electrodiagnostic studies can be helpful in defining the problem in certain instances.

In early cases, night splinting (see Ch. 3) with the wrist in neutral or slight extension may be quite effective. Injection of a steroid-lidocaine combination may be useful both diagnostically and therapeutically, but extreme care must be taken to avoid impaling the nerve. The injection should be made in the ulnar side of the carpal tunnel (Fig. 47) starting at the level of the wrist flexion crease very close to the PL tendon. If paresthesias are elicited, the needle should be withdrawn and reinserted, more ulnar. It is important that the injection be juxtaneural not intraneural. The technique is similar to that for a median nerve block. A total of 2 ml of solution should be used, 1 ml of a steroid and 1 ml of lidocaine.

Definitive treatment is surgical decompression of the carpal tunnel often combined with median neurolysis. This may be done under local or regional anesthesia and is best done in an operating room to ensure sterility and adequate light and instruments. To release the nerve, an incision is made in the midproximal palm up to the wrist level. If the incision needs to be extended proximally, it is turned toward the ulnar side to avoid the palmar cutanoous branch of the median nerve. The palmar fascia is incised, and the nerve is identified just above the carpal canal. A closed hemostat is used to identify the opening of the carpal tunnel, and the transverse carpal ligament is incised from proximal to distal while very carefully observing that the nerve is not injured. Special care must be taken to avoid the motor branch which comes off in a radial palmar direction near the terminal arborization of the nerve. The superficial transverse vascular arch, which lies at the distal end of the carpal canal, must be looked for and not injured.

High median nerve compression

Compression of the median nerve may also occur at various sites high in the forearm. In these cases nonfunction or marked weakness of one or more of the median innervated extrinsic muscles is present (usually the FPL and FDP of the index), and the sensory loss in the hand is less clearly defined or not present.

Ulnar nerve compression

Ulnar nerve compression is uncommon at the wrist level because the ulnar nerve passes into the hand through Guyon's canal, which does not contain any synovium. However, the nerve may be compressed by either thrombosis or aneurysm of the ulnar artery, repetitive trauma to the palm (hypothenar hammer syndrome), anterior dislocation of the ulnar head, or a ganglion arising from the pisohamate joint. Treatment of an ulnar nerve problem in this area is usually surgical.

Compression of the nerve at the elbow (cubital tunnel syndrome) is seen fairly often. This may be caused by a single direct blow on the elbow or may arise as a consequence of chronic mild pressure on this area. The symptoms are numbness in the ulnar half of the ring and the entire small fingers on both the palmar and dorsal aspects as well as weakness of the interossei, AdP, FCU, and FDP to ring and small fingers. To test for ulnar innervated intrinsics have the patient actively cross his fingers or abduct and adduct them. These actions require function of the ulnar innervated interossei muscles.

Effective primary treatment is simple padding of the elbow to avoid compression of the nerve when the patient leans on the elbow. Definitive treatment is surgical release and rerouting of the nerve. Surgery is done under high regional or general anesthesia. The nerve is identified in the cubital tunnel and carefully isolated. Particular care must be taken not to disturb the branches to the flexors, which arise just distal to the elbow. The nerve is then transferred anterior to the medial epicondyle and may be fixed there by any one of several techniques.

Radial nerve compression

The radial nerve may be compressed at the midhumeral level by prolonged pressure causing a neurapraxia manifested by the inability to extend the wrist and the fingers at the MCP joints. Thumb extension at the IP joint will usually be present by virtue of the thumb intrinsic muscles but will not be as strong or complete as normally. There may also be numbness on the radial dorsal aspect of the hand, but this is not as troubling as the motor palsy.

Motor paresis of this nerve can come from a variety of causes including fracture of the humerus, very heavy use of the triceps, or a closed crush injury or prolonged pressure. Perhaps the most common variety is the so-called Saturday night palsy. The name comes from one mechanism of injury, namely compression of the radial nerve at the midhumeral level in a person so deeply intoxicated as to be nearly comatose. In this condition, the person does not move and the steady, prolonged pressure on the nerve is sufficient to render it neurapraxic for periods of several weeks. Spontaneous recovery is usually complete in about 4 weeks. If the palsy persists beyond that, an electromyogram (EMG) and nerve conduction study should be done. The patient is made much more comfortable and functional by using a cock-up wrist splint, which allows the fingers to function fairly well by means of the intrinsic muscles. The splint should be regularly removed for hygiene and passive exercises.

THE ARTHRITIDES

The two most common types of chronic arthritis are rheumatoid arthritis and osteoarthritis.

Rheumatoid arthritis is the prototype of the synovial proliferative type and, in the hand, usually begins with stiff, swollen, painful wrist and finger joints. Dorsal wrist synovitis is often a prominent feature. Patients often have or have had trigger fingers, wrist tenosynovitis, extensor tendon ruptures, and carpal tunnel syndrome. Intrinsic muscles may become fibrotic and shorten. The test for intrinsic tightness is performed by passively holding the patient's MCP joints extended and either actively or passively flexing the IP joints. Since the intrinsics are put on stretch by MCP extension, if they are tight, the IP joints will have limited flexion. With progression of the disease, the digits often become deformed with classic ulnar drift and extensor lag at the MCP joints as well as either swan-neck (hyperextension at the PIP joint and a droop at the DIP joint) or boutonnière (a flexion deformity at the

PIP joint with hyperextension at the DIP joint) deformities at the PIP joints. Radiographs taken early in the disease show periarticular erosions, notably in the metacarpal heads. Later, the radiographs will show loss of the articular surfaces of the bones, and even, loss of bone stock (e.g., total collapse of the carpal bones).

Differential diagnosis of early rheumatoid synovitis of the finger joints includes infection (especially gonococcal), gout, pseudo gout, and acute calcific tendonitis. Initial treatment of the disease is nonsurgical and consists of splinting, therapy, patient education, and various medications. This is a systemic disease and is best managed using a team approach, the team being headed by an interested family physician, internist, or rheumatologist.

In the early phases of the disease the surgeon cannot offer the patient too much. However, dorsal tenosynovectomy done at the proper time can prevent extensor tendon rupture. There is tendency for the synovitis to recur from small remnants that are invariably not excised, so simple synovectomy without medical treatment is not advised. As the disease progresses and deformities appear, joint replacement at wrist, MCP, and PIP joints should be considered. Arthroplasty is combined with soft tissue releases and reconstruction. Postoperatively dynamic splinting and a therapy program are essential. Arthrodesis of various joints can be helpful. The surgeon must always bear in mind that a deformed functional hand is better than a cosmetic nonfunctional one. Therefore a careful evaluation of how the patient uses the hand is very important before any surgery is done on a rheumatoid patient.

Degenerative arthritis or osteoarthritis usually involves the distal digital joints and thumb basal (trapeziometacarpal) joint but may also involve PIP joints. MCP and wrist joints are less commonly involved. The marginal osteophytes at the DIP joints known as Heberden's nodes and those at the PIP joints known as Bouchard's nodes are characteristic of this disease. Small cysts known as mucous cysts may be seen arising from the dorsal aspect of the distal joints. They are a type of ganglion and may cause a grooving of the nail. Surgical excision is usually the best treatment. When excision is done, the surgery is performed under digital block anesthesia. A small ellipse of skin is excised and the lesion traced into the joint. The offending osteophyte should be snipped off with a fine rongeur. Direct closure is almost always possible; if not, a small split thickness skin graft can be used as described in the section on finger pad injuries (see Ch. 6).

The other common site for degenerative arthritis is the thumb basal joint. Patients complain of pain on use of the thumb in a variety of activities. Axial compression of the metacarpal upon the trapezium gives a grinding sensation and is painful. The thumb often has an adducted stance with a prominent "knob" at the basal joint, adduction of the metacarpal, and hyperextension of the MCP joint. It must be differentiated from deQuervain's (see above). The radiograph will show degeneration of the articular surfaces of the trapezium and usually a subluxation of the metacarpal off the trapezium with a characteristic adduction stance.

Treatment of basal joint arthrosis or arthritis in early stages can be with nonsteroidal anti-inflammatory drugs (NSAIDs). Steroid injections occasionally give short-term relief. A "C" splint to hold the thumb web open may give some relief. A variety of surgical procedures including fusion of the joint, implant arthroplasty of various types, and simple trapezium removal with placement of a space filling autogenous tendon are available for long-term relief of severely involved joints.

Traumatic arthritis occurs as a consequence of open or closed trauma. Clinically the patient will complain of marked stiffness and often of considerable pain. Radiographically, marked joint narrowing is seen. Conservative measures include the use of anti-inflammatory drugs, steroid injections, static and dynamic splints, and the various therapy modalities. In this situation, as well as in other problems with chronic stiffness, a good hand therapy program supervised by either an occupational or physical therapist with a special interest in the hand can be of inestimable value. In those patients not responding to conservative treatment, the same operative alternatives can be offered to the patient as for osteoarthritis.

8

THE ROLE OF HAND THERAPY

The ultimate goal of treatment for any hand injury is good function. Initially, healing and stability are important. It is essential to remember, however, that normal hand function requires not only stability but maximum flexibility and good sensibility.

The process of healing may compromise hand flexibility. A combination of immobilization, edema, and scar formation can be deleterious to the hand because of the stiffness that may result. Even a minor injury, when followed by a prolonged period of swelling, may require months of intensive therapy to regain fair hand function. Worse yet, deformity and pain may render a patient unable to return to a former occupation. To minimize such problems, those physicians and other medical personnel treating patients with injured hands should be aware of the potential for such progression of events in an injured hand.

THE EFFECTS OF INJURY

Initially edema is a normal response to injury. An inflammatory phase predictably occurs. This is followed by absorption of extracellular fluid through venous and lymphatic systems and by scar formation. However, dependency, injury to these vessels, nonfunctioning muscles that ordinarily aid flow in the vessels, external compression from constrictive clothing and/or jewelry, inadequate elevation, and overuse of an injured hand can all prevent absorption of edema fluid and cause chronic swelling.

CONSEQUENCES OF EDEMA

Edema may cause tissue necrosis by interfering with both arterial inflow and, more commonly, venous drainage. Additionally, unabsorbed edema fluid may produce abnormally large amounts of scar tissue. The pressure and discomfort caused by the edema may also limit the

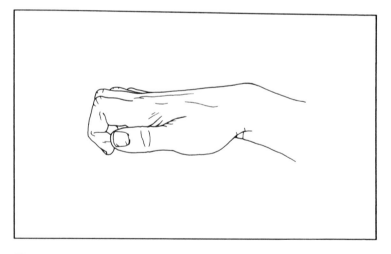

Figure 48
The position of nonfunction, also known as the position of rest-injury, is not acceptable

active motion that is necessary to prevent the formation of scar adhesions. Scar contraction then occurs with joint stiffness, fixation, and deformity. Sometimes pain accompanies this process and contributes to a cycle that eventually ends with the hand in the position of nonfunction (Fig. 48).

PREVENTING NONFUNCTION

Immobilization

Most injured hands need some immobilization to give the tissues a chance to recover. This should be appropriate to the injury in question both in degree and length of time. Only those parts that require immobilization for proper healing should be included in the splint. Other parts

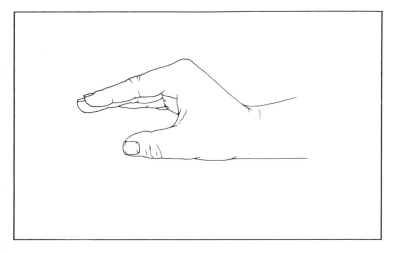

Figure 49
The intrinsic plus or protected position

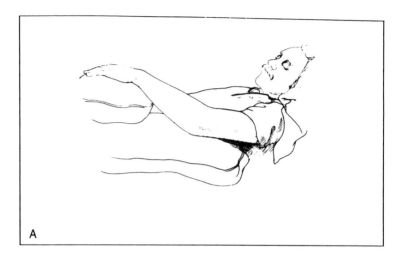

A

should be allowed to move freely to prevent unnecessary stiffness from occurring. Tight proximal constriction must be avoided whether from dressings, jewelry, or clothing. This is especially important in the older patient, who may be more prone to swelling and stiffness, and in persons whose hands are naturally tight and stiff. Short arm splints should be fabricated to allow MCP joint motion and leave the thenar eminence unencumbered (see Ch. 3).

The hand should be immobilized in such a way that it is least likely to stiffen into a position of nonfunction. The wrist should be positioned in 30° to 35° of extension, the MCP joints in 45° to 70° of flexion, the IPs in a slightly flexed (10°) position and the thumb web open (see Figs. 15 and 49). This position is variously called the intrinsic plus position or the protected position.

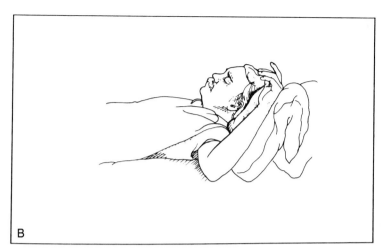

B

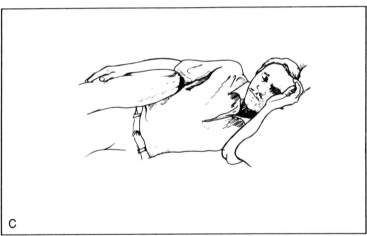

C

Figure 50 (A-C)
Hand positions for sleep

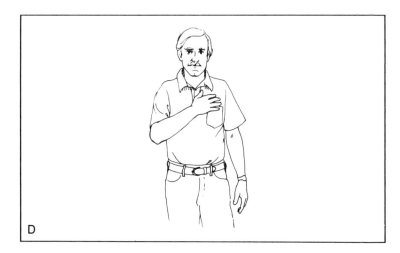

Figure 50
(D) Self-elevation position while standing or walking

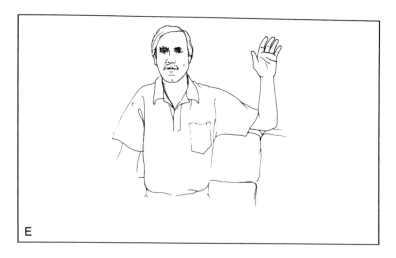

Figure 50
(E) Elevation while sitting

Instructions to the patient

Elevation

The patient must be instructed to hold the hand at heart level or higher until the swelling has disappeared. When the patient can make a full fist and see the wrinkles on the dorsum of the hand, the swelling is gone. Patients should be instructed about proper elevation of the hand when sleeping, walking, and sitting (Figs. 50A-50E). A sling may be a useful device to assist the patient with elevation (see Ch. 3 and Figs. 20, 22A and 22B). However, if it is worn constantly, especially by older patients, marked elbow and shoulder stiffness may develop. It is very disheartening to patient, doctor, and therapist to see the hand fully recover but for the patient to end up with a stiff, painful shoulder. At least three to four times a day on a regular schedule the patient should remove the sling and put the shoulder and elbow through a full ROM. Care should be taken to make sure that the sling really does hold the hand at heart level or higher (see Fig. 19) and not at umbilicus level as is so often the case.

Exercise

Gentle exercises should be prescribed. They should be performed four to five times per day for short periods of time. Exercises should not cause increased swelling or marked pain. They should not necessitate the use of pain medication or cause sleeplessness. Exercises should be performed slowly, gently, and repeatedly until maximum motion is attained (Figs. 51A-51D).

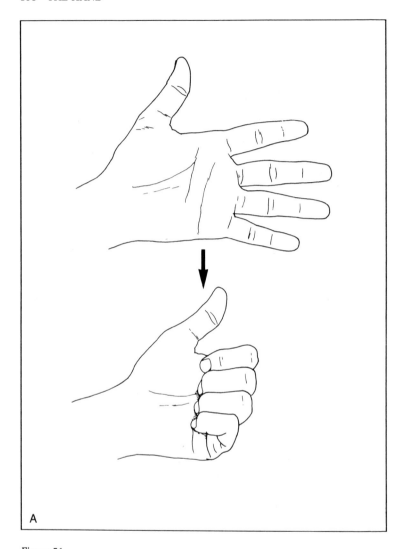

A

Figure 51
(A) Active hand exercises — extension-flexion of the digits to the palmar creases

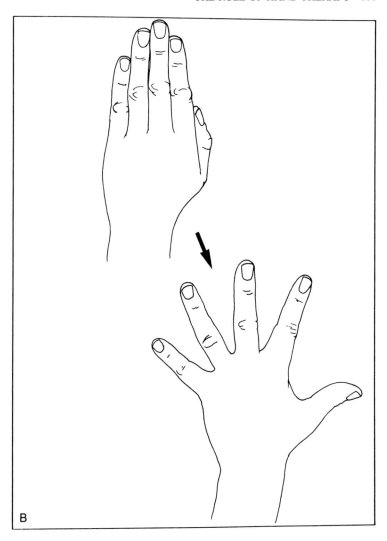

Figure 51
(B) Adduction-abduction of the fingers

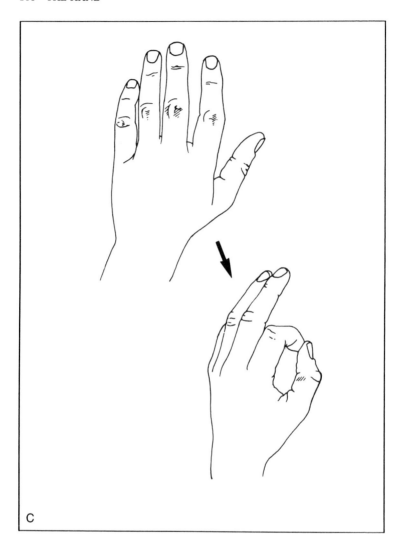

C

Figure 51
(C) Opposition of the thumb to each of the other digits

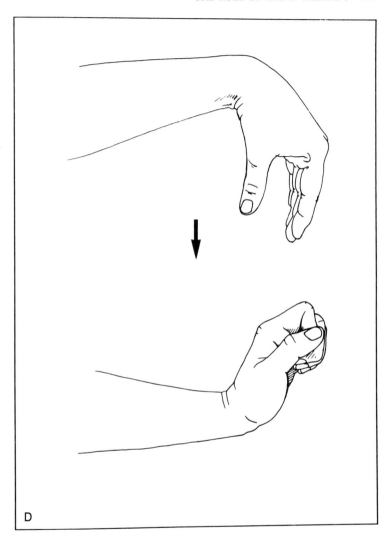

Figure 51
(D) Extension-flexion of the wrist

Soaks

Both warm water soaks and alternate warm-cool soaks may be indicated as a comfort measure. The soaks may be done before or after exercise or exercise may be done while the hand is soaking. A mild detergent can be added to the water to assist in cleansing the wound and skin that has been covered up for several weeks. If possible use a container large enough and deep enough to contain the entire hand and forearm (Fig. 52) in a horizontal or slightly elevated position. Soaking in a dependent position may increase swelling. Warm soak water should be about 100° F. Many patients think that very hot water is best but in fact it increases swelling (and pain). As with exercises, frequent short soaks are better than one prolonged soak. If for any reason soaks increase pain, they should be stopped.

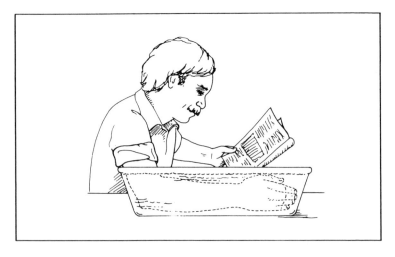

Figure 52
Soaking the injured hand

Referral to hand therapy

Even after receiving the optimal operative and post-operative care, some patients may require a more formal hand rehabilitation program. Not all patients regain maximal or even functional hand use by following the principles outlined above. Some patients do not have the self-discipline required to do these things. In some the severity or complexity of the injury or disease may make doing these things alone difficult or impossible. Some have little desire to recover from an injury that is allowing them paid time-off from a job they do not like. Patients who fall into any of these categories may benefit greatly from formal hand therapy.

An increasing number of therapy departments have registered occupational or physical therapists who have the interest, training, and ability to treat the special needs of patients with hand problems. A hand therapist can provide the patient with an individualized, closely supervised program of exercise, dynamic splinting, muscle and sensory re-education, pain control, work readiness skills, and psychological support to regain good hand function.

If travel distance prohibits therapy on a frequent basis, even periodic therapy sessions of thorough patient education in a home program of proper exercise and splint use may result in great improvement of hand function. The referral to therapy should include a description of the injury and surgery and the need for any precautions. Early intervention by the therapist can often prevent considerable late nonfunction.

Perhaps most important is that the patient become involved in his own rehabilitation. The hand injury has not been fully treated until maximal functional recovery has been achieved.

SUGGESTED READINGS

American Society for Surgery of the Hand: The Hand: Examination and Diagnosis. 3rd. Ed. Churchill Livingstone, New York, 1990

Ariyan S: The Hand Book. 2nd. Ed. Williams & Wilkins, Baltimore, 1983

Beasley RW: Hand Injuries. WB Saunders, Philadelphia, 1981

Boswick JA, Jr: Current Concepts in Hand Surgery. Lea & Febiger, Philadelphia, 1983

Boswick JA, Jr: Complications in Hand Surgery. WB Saunders, Philadelphia, 1986

Boyes JH: Bunnell's Surgery of the Hand. 5th. Ed. JB Lippincott, Philadelphia, 1970

Buck-Gramcko D, Hoffman R, Neumann R: Hand Trauma. A Practical Guide. Thieme, New York, 1986

Burton RI: The hand. p. 273. In Evarts MC (ed): Surgery of the Musculoskeltal System. 2nd. Ed. Churchill Livingstone, New York, 1990

Cailliet R: Hand Pain and Impairment. 3rd. Ed. FA Davis, Philadelphia, 1982

Carter PR: Common Hand Injuries and Infections: A Practical Approach to Early Treatment. WB Saunders, Philadelphia, 1983

Chase RA: Atlas of Hand Surgery. Vol. 1. WB Saunders, Philadelphia, 1973

Chase RA: Atlas of Hand Surgery. Vol. 2. WB Saunders, Philadelphia, 1983

Conolly WB: Color Atlas of Hand Conditions. Yearbook Medical Publishers, Chicago, 1980

Conolly WB, Kilgore ES, Jr: Hand Injuries and Infections. Yearbook Medical Publishers, Chicago, 1979

Flatt AE: The Care of Minor Hand Injuries. 3rd. Ed. CV Mosby, St. Louis, 1972

Flatt AE: Care of the Arthritic Hand. 4th. Ed. CV Mosby, St. Louis, 1983

Flynn JE: Hand Surgery. 3rd. Ed. Williams & Wilkins, Baltimore, 1982

Green DP: Operative Hand Surgery. 2nd. Ed. Churchill Livingstone, New York, 1988

Hunter JM, Schneider LH, Mackin EJ, Callahan AD: Rehabilitation of the Hand. 2nd. Ed. CV Mosby, St. Louis, 1984

Kilgore ES, Jr, Graham WP III: The Hand: Surgical and Nonsurgical Management. Lea & Febiger, Philadelphia, 1977

Lamb DW, Hooper G: Hand Conditions. Churchill Livingstone, Edinburgh, 1984

Lamb DW, Hooper G, Kuczynski MB: The Practice of Hand Surgery. 2nd. Ed. Blackwell Scientific, Boston, 1988

Lampe EW: Surgical anatomy of the hand. CIBA Clin Symp 40(3):1, 1988

Lister G: The Hand: Diagnosis and Indications. 2nd. Ed. Churchill Livingstone, Edinburgh, 1984

Littler JW: The Hand and Upper Extremity. Vol. VI. In Converse JM (ed): Reconstructive Plastic Surgery. 2nd. Ed. WB Saunders, Philadelphia, 1977

Lucas GL: Examination of the Hand. Charles C Thomas, Springfield, IL, 1972

Macnicol MF, Lamb DW: Basic Care of the Injured Hand. Churchill Livingstone, Edinburgh, 1984

Mann RJ: Infections of the Hand. Lea & Febiger, Philadelphia, 1988

Milford L: The Hand. 3rd. Ed. CV Mosby, St. Louis, 1988

Newmeyer WL: Primary Care of Hand Injuries. Lea & Febiger, Philadelphia, 1979

Omer GE, Jr, Spinner M: Management of Peripheral Nerve Problems. WB Saunders, Philadelphia, 1980

Sandzen SC, Jr: Atlas of Wrist and Hand Fractures. PSG Publishing, Littleton, MA, 1979

Sandzen SC, Jr: Atlas of Acute Hand Injuries. McGraw-Hill, New York, 1980

Schamber D: Simply Performed Tests of the Hand. Vantage Press, New York, 1984

Semple C: The Primary Management of Hand Injuries. Yearbook Medical Publishers, Chicago, 1979

Spinner M: Injuries to the Major Branches of Peripheral Nerves of the Forearm. 2nd. Ed. WB Saunders, Philadelphia, 1978

Spinner M: Kaplan's Functional and Surgical Anatomy of the Hand. 3rd. Ed. JB Lippincott, Philadelphia, 1984

Strickland JW, Steichen JB: Difficult Problems in Hand Surgery. CV Mosby, St. Louis, 1982

Tubiana R, Thomine JM, Mackin E: Examination of the Hand and Upper Limb. WB Saunders, Philadelphia, 1984

Weckesser EC: Treatment of Hand Injuries: Preservation and Restoration of Function. Yearbook Medical Publishers, Chicago, 1974

Weeks PM, Wray RC: Management of Acute Hand Injuries. CV Mosby, St. Louis, 1978

Wolfert FG: Acute Hand Injuries — A Multispecialty Approach. Little Brown, Boston, 1980

Wynn-Parry CB: Rehabilitation of the Hand. 4th. Ed. Butterworth, Woburn, MA, 1981

Index

Page numbers followed by *f* indicate figures; those followed by *t* indicate tables.